Pathways through Pain

Pathways through Pain

Women's Journeys

ANN CALLENDER

Foreword by the Rt Revd Lord Runcie

THE PILGRIM PRESS
Cleveland, Ohio

The Pilgrim Press
Cleveland, Ohio 44115

Copublished with Darton, Longman and Todd Ltd
London, England

© 1999 Ann Callender
Foreword © 1999 Robert Runcie

Bible quotations are taken from the Revised English Bible,
© 1989 Oxford University Press and Cambridge University Press.

Printed and bound in Great Britain.

04 03 02 01 00 99   5 4 3 2 1

Library of Congress Cataloging-in-Publication Data

Callender, Ann.
    Pathways through pain : women's journeys / Ann Callender.
      p. cm.
    Includes bibliographical references.
    ISBN 0-8298-1306-3 (pbk. : alk. paper)
    1. Chronic pain–Patients–Religious life. 2. Callender, Ann.
   3. Chronic pain–Religious aspects–Christianity. 4. Women mystics.
I. Title.
BV4910.335.C35   1999
248.8'6–dc21   98-54172
                                         CIP

For
Canon Richard Buck and
The Revd Dr Victoria Raymer

Contents

Foreword

IT IS HARD to think of anyone who would not feel better for reading this book. It is an understated gem. Part of the reason is that Ann Callender can write with such clarity and grace. We are never at the mercy of devotional clichés nor does she drift off into abstractions. She has a story to tell of her own life of chronic pain and the way in which a traditional Christian faith has enabled her to live with it. The mixture of biography, spiritual insight and fascinating historical narrative works brilliantly. Digressions never get out of hand but they serve to reduce any intensity and open out the main issue to those who simply want to live an authentic Christian life.

Ann disclaims any spectacular or heroic scale in her ordeals though she made me shiver at the way she poked scissors into her right eye when she was five and took a full-powered baseball hit which shattered her knee when she was twelve. She lives every day with the consequences of both. She shows herself brisk and cheerful in the world as an attractive wife and mother. A lighter touch here and there displays that humour which she regards as essential for a proper perspective on life from those who are all too prone to self-pity. At the same time there is an impressive reticence about the horrors which have too often been her own lot in life. This kind of distinction between humour on the outskirts of religion and sensitivity to senseless tragedy is important. She understands it, indeed takes it for granted.

The author states at the beginning that she is not a theologian or philosopher. Certainly this is not a book which deals with 'The Problem of Pain'. Nor are there any technical terms which are common to those who juggle with ideas. Theology is not to be confined to the problem-solving of professional academics. Augustine in his Confessions as in his writings on the Trinity is discovering the truth within himself. So too with Jesus. The appeal of his teaching was that every word of it had been lived, and because Jesus also conveyed truth by parables he avoided stuffing things down people's throats. So there is the highest authority for the theology that you find in this book. Hence too the spiritual refreshment and nourishment that it offers.

The Rt Revd and Rt Hon. Lord Runcie of Cuddesdon
Archbishop of Canterbury 1980–91

Introduction

I HAVE written this book in the first place to answer a personal question, and in the second to share that answer with those in a predicament similar to mine. I am an ordinary Christian living in ordinary pain. That is to say, I am a reasonably faithful follower of Christ who copes daily with the quite unspectacular kind of pain which millions of other people suffer. Occasionally, the pain becomes unbearable. Generally, however, it remains contained and endurable with little outward sign of distress. Most of the time struggling with it is a very private affair, one I share with God but otherwise try to keep to myself. How best to live with it and grow through it – rather than be diminished by it – have been the questions of a lifetime.

In the search for answers I turned to the saints for guidance. Many of the valiant souls formally labelled as saints encountered horrific pain on their road to holiness and heaven. Many more Christians, who have led less conspicuous if no less heroic lives of sanctity, have also endured considerable suffering. From the first group I have chosen St Teresa of Avila and St Thérèse of Lisieux and from the second group a wide selection of courageous but less well-known individuals. Each confronted very different kinds of pain in vastly different circumstances. Nevertheless, all grew into the full stature of their sanctified being through the experience of suffering.

I have studied the saints' ways of dealing with pain and tried to make sense of them in terms of my own experience. I have striven to do so with humility, recognising that the pain endured by many of the saints has been far more intense than mine and that the wisdom and fortitude of the saints has been far greater than my own. Nevertheless, I hope that observations from a more modest perspective will offer particular help to those whose pain is also less dramatic and whose spiritual experiences are less exalted. To convey these insights I have chosen the historical approach rather than the scriptural for two reasons. First, by training and profession I am an historian, not a theologian, and as a consequence I am more adept at analysing people's lives than at explaining Scripture. Second, I regard the saints' stories as compelling illustrations of faith-in-practice and as examples of holy living worthy of study and emulation.

Before recounting their gripping stories, allow me briefly to relate how I know personally about chronic pain and disability. My first encounter with suffering occurred when I was five years old. One Sunday morning before church, while using my mother's sharp sewing scissors to cut an intricate costume for a paper doll, I poked the shears into my right eye. Surgery was discussed but rejected. Instead, eye exercises and a patch over the good eye were prescribed for several years in an attempt to restore the use of the damaged eye. Neither was successful and 'lazy-eyed blindness' persisted. Like any child, I accepted the abnormal as normal and felt no sense of disability. My family alternately joked and despaired at my propensity to collide with – and often break – objects which I could not see on my right, while my friends laughed about the hideous black patch and called me 'Hopalong' after the one-eyed star of a cowboy programme on children's television. Otherwise, the eye problem was ignored by me and by everyone around me.

Visual impairment contributed to the second source of suffering. At the age of twelve I was standing on the third base line while watching an American baseball game when the batter hit a foul ball and I, not seeing it coming, received its full force (the equivalent of a six in cricket) on my right knee. It shattered. Six operations followed over the next fifteen years while osteoarthritis settled not only in that knee, but in other joints as well. Despite the predictions of several orthopaedists that I would be crippled by middle age, I can still move about with relative ease most of the time. Because I have displayed my difficulties at home rather than at work, most of my friends and colleagues are unaware of my predicament. I freely expose my vulnerabilities to them so that I may share some of the lessons I have learned over forty years with those in similar circumstances.

It follows that some of the chapters of this book will be historical and others autobiographical. I have mixed the two in order to supply a personal comment on each historical section. The result of this combination of historical and personal is an alternation of style between the scholarly and the chatty, the dispassionate and the intimate. I hope that this alternation in subject and tone does not prove disruptive. It is the only means I could find to make this book accessible to those who wish to explore their suffering and find ways of coping with it inside the wider context of the Christian tradition and beside a fellow sufferer who has lived and grown through a lifetime of pain.

To present this material I have employed the analogy of a journey. I believe that our lives are adventures which begin at birth and extend into eternity. Along the way opportunities arise to make a choice of direction. Some paths will lead us forward to discover new talents, to form new and deeper relationships with each other and with God, and to advance towards the heavenly vision of lasting peace and joy. Others will draw us into sterile activities, dysfunctional relationships and abiding disappointment.

The aim of this book is to chart various journeys taken by Christian men and women over the past two thousand years and to distinguish between the creative and the destructive. I begin with my own personal itinerary, as I have ventured some way down all of the paths described in this book and can testify to their utility or futility. Next, I shall examine pathways which have led to a healthy integration of mind, body and spirit. These include routes taken by Jesus, St Paul, the martyrs and religious. Then I shall analyse two pathways which have led to even greater suffering – the denial of pain through dualist systems like Christian Science and the distortion of pain through masochism. Finally, I shall tell the stories of two remarkable women who used their experiences of pain to endow their lives with rich meaning.

In writing and researching this book I am greatly indebted to friends who have supplied information, offered encouragement and given sound advice. Without the prompting of two of my oldest friends – the Revd Dr Victoria Raymer and Canon Richard Buck – I would never have begun this project, let alone completed it. They have been unfailingly supportive and have given unstintingly of their time, their books and their wisdom. Prebendary John Gaskell has carefully read, marked and criticised every chapter so that the book is far shorter and much improved through his querying and slashing. William Vollmer and Dr Michael Berg have tutored me in topics relating to psychiatric and psychological problems, and Dr Maurice Lipsedge has supplied invaluable articles and welcome encouragement. Miss Jane Wakefield has offered the perspective of a fellow traveller and has made useful suggestions about signposting the terrain of pain. Miss Rosemary Goad has given wise counsel at critical moments. Sr Margaret Anne ASSP has provided guidance and help with proofreading. Finally, the All Saints Sisters of the Poor have extended abundant hospitality, years of practical and prayerful support and a haven in which to write. To all who have assisted me so generously in so many ways, I offer my heartfelt thanks. For all errors I accept full and singular responsibility.

All Saints Convent
Oxford
July 1998

Chapter One

My Itinerary

I SET OFF on my journey through pain on the wrong route. I pursued that path for nearly fifteen years. It was a disaster. Because I was too proud to accept that my gut reaction to pain was fear, I stalwartly refused to face my fear and became as crippled by it as by the arthritis. Had I displayed the honesty and courage to face my terror of pain and of the road ahead, I could have launched my journey towards creative suffering far sooner. Failing to do so, I wandered into cul-de-sacs which led to frustration, anxiety and even more pain. Avoiding this kind of pointless meandering entails confronting your fear without shame or embarrassment and realising that it is an altogether natural and spontaneous response which we share with the lower animals. They remain ever reactive and ever frightened. Many of us do too. The essential first step towards creative suffering is to quell the fear by acknowledging pain as an unwelcome yet inescapable part of your life. Only then can you begin to discover its potential as an agent of construction rather than destruction.

In my experience there are two basic kinds of fear: a fear of the physical pain and also an existential fear arising from that physical suffering. The physical sort has three varieties. The first is of low intensity but long duration. It is best described as a dull ache – for me, the feeling of a heavy weight pressing on sore joints during waking hours and sometimes interrupting sleep as well. It is most noticeable first thing in the morning, late in the day after long committee meetings, concerts or dinners, and after idiotic attempts to sprint too quickly, stand too long or carry too much. It varies in intensity, but it is almost always there. It saps my energy and ruins my disposition. It is an ordinary, everyday variety of chronic pain. It makes movement difficult, but it does not entirely disrupt mobility or thought. I can move about and think over it. Indeed, displacing my attention and changing position are the most positive ways of dealing with it and living through it. In this kind of pain I can pretend to others that all is well and I am 'normal'. But it isn't and I'm not. It depletes my energy while I carry on with everyday activities. At the office I can and do maintain a calm disposition, but at home I sometimes let the mask slip. At bad moments any request from my nearest and dearest to undertake an extra chore or respond to family needs can crack the surface of equanimity and expose the tension of coping with pain and life's usual litany of responsibilities simultaneously.

For years my husband has complained of the sergeant-major tone of voice I adopt when the pain level rises and those at home do not perform as I desire or expect. For years my biggest challenge has been to adopt a more conciliatory manner. After much striving I have learned to keep my frustrations to myself most of the time. I have changed the way I deal with the pain, the tension, myself and others, but I cannot eliminate the ache. This kind of pain is ever with me, slowly worsening over time. I am frightened by it. And insofar as fear is rational, I would be foolish not to be afraid, for it potentially destroys the quality of the day for myself and those I love most.

The second type of pain comes in a sudden, intense flash. It is like a double-edged knife jab, cutting across nerves and briefly but powerfully resonating through my entire body. It takes me completely by surprise and makes me jump. It also frightens me. One source of fright is the unpleasantness of the pain itself. A second source of fright is the loss of control which occurs during these attacks. We are all afraid of being ambushed by something sinister. This is the animating force of children's fairy tales and adult horror stories. It evokes an immediate terrified response in all human beings of whatever age or culture. As adults, we are also profoundly disturbed at the prospect of being taken unawares and unprepared by life's litany of real horrors – a terrible car crash, the sudden loss of a child, spouse or partner, the announcement of a terminal disease. These take us by surprise and send us reeling in panic. Equally distressing is the sudden jab of searing pain. It alerts us that we are not in control of events or ourselves. It hurts us physically and embarrasses us socially. Try to continue a conversation or sip a cup of tea during an attack! Both are impossible. The attack strips you of the mask of normality and exposes your total weakness and vulnerability. This kind of pain is entirely upsetting of mind, body and social 'bella figura'. But it is not the worst variety.

The third type of physical pain is the most terrifying. It comes in relentless waves which overwhelm my entire being. Though not necessarily more intense than the second type, it is far more prolonged. Time stops. The pain extends into an eternity. I am immobilised for the duration. Normal bodily rhythms are fractured. I pant because I can neither inhale nor exhale smoothly and deeply. My consciousness is riveted exclusively on the surges of pain which engulf my mind as well as my body. In my experience there is no physical energy or cognitive perspective available to focus on anything else, including God. Perhaps over time I shall grow sufficiently in grace to perceive God as immanent in all events and at all times, even during these excruciating attacks. But I doubt it, not simply because of my personal limitations, but also because of my human ones. Jesus, in far worse pain on the cross, searched for a reassuring sense of God's presence and found none. He cried out, 'My God, my God, why have You forsaken me?' Why should I not also feel abandoned during pain's worst assaults? In these agonising circumstances God is revealed after the event – at Easter for Jesus, and for me in the aftermath of an attack, as I regain physical and mental composure and realise that I have just been drawn more

3

deeply into the mystery of pain, death and ultimate re-creation.

In addition to the various degrees of physical pain is existential pain. This springs from our nature as sentient, cognitive beings. We not only feel the bodily assault; we react to it emotionally as well. Then we think about both the physical and emotional distress in an attempt to understand our experience. The cumulative process produces a pain which envelops our entire selves. I am even more frightened of this kind of pain than the purely physical, because it encompasses the past and future as well as the present by projecting the immediate discomfort on to the scale of a lifetime. It interprets my fate as a human being exclusively in terms of suffering. It is utterly unmanageable and terrifying.

As with physical pain, there are three facets of existential pain. For me the first arises from a fear of disability and immobility. I watch my body slowly deteriorate over the years and my faculty for movement gradually, almost imperceptibly, diminish. When living with the everyday sort of ache, this prospect is of little concern and no real terror. I am inconvenienced but not stopped in my tracks. I climb steps one at a time, but I reach the top. I awaken when I roll over at night, but I nonetheless usually obtain a reasonable rest. It is only when the two more ferocious types of pain assault me that my perspective blurs and I stare at a vision of immobility. Rationally, I counsel myself to remain calm and focus on the present moment. I force myself to rehearse the number of times I have been warned of impending doom and it has not come – yet. But lingering at the back of my mind is the memory of being bed-bound, wheelchair bound, and restricted by leg-iron, casts, crutches and sticks. They are all part of my life experience. They are not necessarily relegated to the past. They could easily be part of the future. So my fears are not unfounded. They are legitimate.

The second kind of existential pain relates to my character. I am frightened that it will degenerate under the stress of protracted pain and that I will become someone I do not wish to be – a gorgon of pessimism and bad temper. Like anyone else in chronic discomfort, I routinely become disheartened and occasionally depressed by the relentless nature of the pain. During these low moods my patience with myself and others evaporates. At home my tone becomes acerbic. I seem to become ever more tired and ever more irritable. I fully comprehend St Paul's lament that 'the good which I want to do, I fail to do. . . . When I want to do the right, only the wrong is within my reach' (Romans 7:19, 21). Remembering episodes of brittle disposition in the past and anticipating a future of waning patience and good humour, I become discouraged, angry and self-pitying.

There is only one state worse than this. It is the sense of, and fear of, isolation. During pain's fiercest assaults – which mercifully have not occurred for quite a few years – I have retreated into myself. I have been unable to communicate with anyone because my attention has been sharply focused on surviving the onslaughts of acute pain in as dignified a fashion as possible. There has been no energy left for normal concerns or conversations. During these agonising episodes I have experienced 'separation anxiety', the most intense form of existential pain. I have felt cut off not only from other people, but also from God as well. This sense of ultimate and complete isolation has been my experience of hell on earth.

Enduring these varying kinds and degrees of pain without being disfigured and perhaps even destroyed by them has necessitated finding a framework of meaning through which to interpret them. I, personally, could not live with any of this pain unless I were a Christian. I could not survive unless I believed that at some profound, usually unperceived level, God is making something positive of the suffering. Exactly what is being created has yet to be revealed. It may be my transformed, sanctified being. It may have little or nothing to do with me personally. It may benefit others in particular or the cosmos in general. I do not know, and I do not need to know.

But I do need to believe that good is somehow being worked out of these struggles which so often seem only to portend destruction. Similarly, I find it essential to believe that the Spirit is joining me in the battle, supplying grace to make the best of it. Without this immediate, ongoing source of inspiration and power, I could not withstand the daily aches, the occasional onslaughts of more spectacular pain or the existential anxiety which they create.

It has taken decades for me to appreciate the full impact of pain on my life. As a teenager and young adult, I admitted the problem of mobility and bad temper which pain generated, but I stubbornly refused to face their source, which was the pain itself. With spectacularly misguided optimism and naivety, I reckoned that to ignore the pain, to smile through it and pretend that it did not exist was the most Christian and positive way to deal with it. Hearty cheerfulness became increasingly difficult to sustain as physical problems became more complicated, periods in plaster and on crutches became more frequent, and the pain became more acute. Only after several operations in quick succession in my late teens and early twenties did I begin to question not so much the wisdom of this façade, alas, but how long I could keep it up.

When I was a twenty-five year old graduate student doing research in London on my doctoral dissertation, one of the friends to whom this book is dedicated tried to persuade me of the untenability of my position. Sitting me down with a very tall, very strong gin and tonic, he casually enquired if I were angry about my predicament, and if not, why not. 'No, I am not at all angry', I replied brightly but vehemently. These prescient queries made no sense to me, for I had spent thirteen years buttressing the façade and desperately avoiding acknowledging the pent-up emotions behind it. His questions were simply too threatening to consider.

The discrepancy between appearance and reality widened appreciably in the next few years. On the surface I remained a fully-functioning academic, sustaining a demanding schedule of teaching, writing and travelling, all the while learning new skills in keeping going despite the pain. But beneath the surface the pain mounted as problems grew worse.

From London I set off to India to undertake more research, still grinning despite being encumbered by a leather and metal brace, limping along with hand luggage which was so heavy it bent my crutches and wearing a miniskirt – what a sight! Upon returning to Cambridge, Massachusetts the next year, I had a long operation which created more problems than it solved. Afterwards I gave history tutorials to Harvard and Radcliffe undergraduates while reclining in a semi-prone position. (My mother said I looked like Elizabeth Barrett Browning and only required Flush, the dog, to complete the pathetic scene.) The next year I married my English husband in California while leaning on an orchid-strewn cane. On honeymoon in Hawaii he gallantly carried me up and down stairs and cliffs for convenience and speed, somehow avoiding a hernia. Our happiness was bittersweet, however, for after the honeymoon he returned to London and I remained in California to have a major knee operation. Six months later, hobbling on a stick, I set off for London to start a new life. The pain was more bearable, and the pleasures of marriage and historical research were both numerous and intense. The next twelve months were blissful. A year later, however, my new-found happiness was vanquished by a sixth knee operation and the death of my entire family in California between August and December 1975.

Stripped of the wan smile and false optimism, I faced the lunacy of continued denial. My spirits plummeted and I entered a tunnel of depression. I remained there for a year and a half. In the circumstances of bereavement on this scale, no one regarded my depression as unusual. Few realised that my loss extended beyond my relatives and American home to the imminent loss of mobility which three eminent orthopaedists grimly predicted. Despite the comfort of my new husband and close friends I felt as if I were floundering around in hell.

During these eighteen months I played unprofitable games to minimise the devastating emotional impact of this newly-accepted inner reality. The worst was an attempt to embrace fatalism. I reasoned that since degeneration was inevitable, hope was misplaced and even counterproductive. 'Accept the unacceptable now,' I told myself, 'and avoid continuing disappointment as the joints deteriorate.' For six months I tried very hard to maintain this apparently sane solution, but I was miserable. Life without hope was life without a future and without joy. A true Stoic might have been able to maintain this sensible if dismal posture, but I could not. My innate optimism asserted itself. I realised that I could not survive without the vision of a viable future, however inappropriate that image might seem. Witness those who hope against hope in the face of terminal illness and even imminent death. They are not being fools. They are being deeply human, displaying an abiding need to look forward to a better tomorrow. Even in ordinary chronic pain and in interludes of more intense pain, I discovered this basic hope to be essential.

Recognising at last that I could neither avoid nor diminish the physical and emotional experience of pain, I determined to find a way to accept it, to be honest and realistic yet hopeful. As a Christian, I turned to the church and discovered a new depth and meaning in the sacraments. Several years earlier – during the chat over the stiff gin and tonic – I had acknowledged that I needed help with the pain. Dimly, I had then perceived that somehow God and I were in this struggle together and that his grace would come to my rescue if I but sought it. I gratefully received the sacrament of healing, an anointing with oil which outwardly and visibly signified the imparting of an inward and spiritual grace. The simple ceremony was deeply moving and consoling. Nevertheless, because I was still denying the extent of my predicament, I failed to derive its full benefit. Only when I finally admitted not only the pain, but also the fears it engendered, did the total impact of the sacrament hit me. Here was a source of power to suffer yet endure, whatever form the pain took and however long the trials.

The sacrament of penance, which I had practised since the age of twenty-one, also took on a vibrant new meaning. Auricular confession provided a regular means of taking stock of my sins of commission (biting off someone's head in frustration, elevating my own selfish desires above the legitimate needs of family and friends, succumbing to the temptations of jealousy or resentment) as well as my numerous sins of omission (not doing what I should have done for a variety of apparently good but actually feeble reasons, elevating my own problems over those of other people and remaining blind to their predicaments). It is immensely liberating to rehearse my worst thoughts and deeds before another person and to be forgiven in the name of God and on behalf of human society. It is obviously not a substitute for apologising to the individuals against whom I have sinned. It is a magnificent supplement. It lifts the burden of failure and frees me from the shackles of the past, enabling me to move forward, to learn from my mistakes and try again and again and again.

A third source of power whose potency I began to appreciate more fully was the eucharist, the Church's celebration of life and death, its foretaste of the heavenly banquet. Frequent communion offered a readily available fount of energy to be used not only to cope with pain, but even more importantly, to fuel all that made life worthwhile for me – love and creativity. Revitalised through the sacrament of healing, restored through the sacrament of penance and reinvigorated by the sacrament of the eucharist, I could live with the pain, not despite it.

Through the sacraments a slow, silent revolution occurred in my experience of pain.[1] I realised that pain was an awkward, permanent, attention-grabbing function of my physical and emotional being. It was part of me, not an alien invader. To interpret it as the enemy and declare war on it was to indulge in a futile civil war with myself. Gradually, I discovered how to

9

befriend it, to relax in its presence, to accommodate it and even to respect it. As the sense of warfare receded, peaceful co-existence developed. I calmed down and cheered up, for I was no longer stifling powerful emotions and fighting against reality. When at the age of thirty-six I returned to Cambridge, Massachusetts on holiday, my former Harvard adviser announced: 'We have never seen you this way.' Truly at ease with myself and life for the first time in over twenty years, I was fully alive. In the next five years I wrote two books, refurbished our house, taught university courses in history, became involved in local politics and charities and had a baby.

In retrospect I understand that the process of accepting pain proceeds through stages which are similar to those of accepting death. Perhaps this is fitting, for one is dying to an existence without pain and physical restrictions and embracing an unchosen life of discomfort and disability. In both situations one is facing the spectre of disintegration – in death of a seemingly total variety, in chronic pain of a less drastic but nonetheless radical sort. The biggest difference between the two is the time framework in which the process occurs. In the face of death the timing is usually concentrated, while in the face of chronic pain it is extended. The timing is different, but the process of accepting one's plight is remarkably similar.

This process has been admirably defined by Elisabeth Kübler-Ross in her seminal and eminently readable book, *On Death and Dying*.[2] The first stage of this process is denial. I sincerely hope that others in chronic pain are faster in passing through this than I was.

The second stage is anger. For me this anger took two forms, one turned inwards as depression and the other outwards in fury at the Almighty. 'How can you do this to me?' I demanded repeatedly. 'If you really want to use me to build your kingdom on earth in my own small way, why are you destroying me?' It took years for me to comprehend that I was asking a different question: 'If you want to use me as *I* think I should be used, why are you doing this to me?' I now understand that I was failing to grasp the fundamental truth that suffering can be a powerful engine of reconstruction. Only when I began asking what God wanted me to be and to become through suffering did the anger abate. I began to surrender my pride and with it the persona which I had so doggedly created over thirty-something years. I began to perceive that God was allowing me to be challenged, broken and remade. There was no place for self-direction or self-glory in this revelation, but rather humility, responsiveness and gratitude. There was also freedom. I surrendered the false pride which prompted the belief that I was in control of my life and was therefore responsible for creating it single-handedly. This was tremendously liberating. Being responsible for life decisions and being responsible for one's ultimate destiny are not at all the same thing. In my experience true freedom arises from appreciating the profound difference.

The last and best consequence of assuaging the anger was peace. As I was growing up, my mother often lamented that I would never know serenity. Suffering from a heart damaged by rheumatic fever as a child but never mentioning it or complaining, she knew all too well the inner emotional turmoil smouldering behind the brave smile. How I wish that she, too, could have admitted her pain to herself and others, shedding a terrible burden of responsibility for that over which she had no control and thus finding inner peace.

The third phase of coming to terms with chronic pain, as with death, is bargaining. Fatalism was one form of bargaining for me. 'If I absolutely give up hope of recovery and totally accept the inevitable right now,' I begged, 'will you leave me alone, and perhaps even let the pain diminish a bit?' This plea did not get any further than a second ruse, a truly embarrassing one. 'Do you suppose that this extended period of suffering will refine me sufficiently for heaven so that little or no time need be spent in the purifying realm of purgatory?' I asked. 'Will I not have earned some reward for all of this pain?' I blush at the sheer brazenness of this entreaty as well as at its

11

glib assumption that I, a mortal, could know what purification and purgatory actually are and that I could accomplish this work on earth. Mercifully, this bargaining stage was for me short-lived.

Acceptance – the fourth and last stage – followed once I discovered the power of the sacraments. Slowly, I began to appreciate the potential for a new persona in Christ being built from the wreckage of my physical and emotional self in a way which was incomprehensible to me and thus totally outside my control. All I had to do was listen to God, allow him to guide me and trust that whatever emerged was roughly what he intended so long as I remained faithful to whatever I discerned from him through prayer and intuition. For a time I begged him to give me a map for the future, a vision of where I was going and who or what I would become. Equipped with such a guide, I could deal with all the variables of life which I found so perplexing to reconcile. Not surprisingly, the Almighty resisted this entreaty. Once again, I had missed the point. Patiently, he led me to realise that in the absence of a map I would have to trust the Mapmaker and follow him day by day as best possible. Only then could my stupendous pride and ego remain disengaged. Only then could I become a new creation in Christ rather than another self-made model of myself.

Since that revelation life has become an adventure. It has had many moments of uncertainty. Through them I have been learning to be courageous in the way Winston Churchill defined the word – displaying grace under pressure. The journey here and into eternity remains an ongoing mystery, but it is not as frightening as it once was. To a degree I can laugh at, with and in the pain. I can also at times appreciate the gifts it brings. One is fellow feeling for others in distress of any sort. Suffering at its deepest level is a common experience with a common vocabulary. Another gift is the freedom to enjoy the passing moment, to take each day as it comes, to be thankful for what is life-affirming and accepting of what is life-denying in it.

I would have preferred to live without pain, but I must acknowledge that its heritage has been generous and immensely valuable. It taught me how to cope with difficult problems as a child and teenager, and to that extent it prepared me to deal with life's struggles earlier than my friends who enjoyed an untroubled childhood and adolescence. It also showed me how to keep going without reference to discomfort, focus my attention sharply and maintain my concentration through virtually any distraction. Over the past forty years the pain has exerted such a powerful influence on my daily life that it has, in many significant ways, made me who I am.

Chapter Two

The Straight Road to Heaven:
The Way of Jesus, St Paul and the Martyrs

CHRISTIANITY teaches us that we exist within an intimate unity of body, emotions and spirit. Most of us accept this proposition as existentially true. Those of us who live in pain are perhaps even more aware of this unity than those who enjoy constant good health. We readily appreciate the intricate relationship between body, emotions and spirit and the need to keep all three in balance. We know from experience that if one part of this triad breaks down, the whole being suffers and illness of one sort or another follows. Thus, a depleted body saps emotions and spirit; ravaged emotions immobilise body and spirit; while a spirit in turmoil wreaks havoc on both body and emotions. Pain is evidence of this breakdown. All of the saints in this study experienced a disintegration of the vital harmony. The causes were different but the result was the same – a collapse of the whole person. For most of them, as for most of us in chronic pain, the source of destruction was apparently external, usually a virus or bacteria, occasionally a genetic defect or accident. For some of them, as for us, it lay hidden in the emotions. Salvation for all came not only from treating the overt disease, but also from restoring the essential internal triad.

The model of Christian health is, of course, Jesus. In the Gospels we encounter a man who maintained an exemplary balance between body, emotions and spirit, a man whose spirit remained ever vibrant, even through the torment of his last twenty-four hours before death. We rightly regard his spiritual integrity as the foundation of his sanctified being, and prayer as both the source and expression of this holiness. From the synoptic Gospels of Matthew, Mark and Luke we also learn much about his emotional vitality. In these books we see him expressing the full range of human emotions – love, anger, pity, compassion, sadness, confusion and even desolation. Further, we witness him displaying tolerance and forgiveness, those spiritual virtues which undergird emotional wellbeing. We watch him accept himself as the son of God as well as the son of Mary and Joseph and accept other people fully and immediately, from prostitutes to tax collectors to aristocratic landowners. We marvel at his ability to forgive others on behalf of God and humanity while pursuing a ministry of reconciliation as the focus of his life's work. Alas, we know nothing of his physical health. But the absence of information about illness suggests a robustness which enabled him to withstand the physical strains of first-century Palestine, where insanitary living conditions, malnutrition and epidemics were common sources of misery and death.

Jesus, himself, may have been healthy in body, emotions and spirit but he did not deny the reality of suffering. Indeed, he deplored pain and sought to vanquish the diseases which caused it. The Gospels abound in healing miracles, instances in which he reversed physical degeneration and even death by invoking divine power to stop a haemorrhage, to rekindle breath or to alleviate emotional anguish by absolving guilt. These books also give weighty evidence to his compassion for those who were anxious for the sick and dying, for those who mourned and for those who were ostracised because of their illnesses. He recognised that pain was the coinage of life. His reaction was to weep about it and to cure it. His own death was excruciating, and through it he validated the physical struggles of his followers through the ages. His resurrection was not just spiritual, but corporal as well. At death his body was changed but not abandoned. The substantial being who appeared to Mary Magdalene on Easter morning, walked with the disciples to Emmaus and ascended forty days later apparently displayed attributes of body, emotion and spirit particular to the man whom they had known as Jesus of Nazareth.

St Paul strove to emulate Jesus and maintain the threefold harmony. He struggled because he lived in chronic pain. He called it the 'thorn in his flesh' (2 Corinthians 12:7). We do not know what exactly it was, for Paul used the word 'flesh' to refer not so much to the body, itself, as to the condition of fallen humanity. His pain may have been physical, but it may equally have been psychological. All we know for certain is that in repeated prayers he begged the Lord to remove it. To his initial dismay the divine answer was a resounding 'no'. Gradually, and perhaps reluctantly, Paul realised that God could use this weakness for his own purpose. Overcoming his gigantic pride, he learned to rely on grace rather than his own stubborn willpower. He accepted this immensely difficult personal challenge and wrote of it to encourage new Christians faced with disease, death and even martyrdom. He assured them that they, and the entire universe, were like a woman giving birth, 'groaning' to bring forth a new creation in and through Christ (Romans 8:22, 25). He inspired them to appreciate pain as a tool for building the heavenly city and fashioning its citizens.

For those to whom St Paul wrote – and for Paul himself – martyrdom was a lively possibility. In some parts of Asia, Africa and South America it remains so today. Martyrdom is the quintessential form of Christian suffering, because it provides the most obvious means of conforming to Christ's own life. It is the true *imitatio Christi*, the most literal way of obeying the Lord's call to 'follow me'. Whereas women have been poorly represented in the ranks of the clergy of all denominations through the ages, they have almost equalled men among the 'noble army of martyrs'. In Greek the word martyr means witness. It has been the role of these women to bear witness to Christ not only by confessing their faith before hostile tribunals, but also by enduring horrendous pain, humiliation and finally death rather than renounce their Saviour.

The possibility of martyrdom first arose within the Jewish communities in which Christianity took root. When Christianity emerged as a gentile religion, the opportunities for martyrdom increased. The Roman authorities sought to eliminate Christianity as a new cult by depriving it of the legal recognition accorded Judaism and by depriving Christians of the toleration extended to Jews who refused to participate in the Roman civic religion. The moment of truth came for Christians when they were required to demonstrate their loyalty to the state by burning incense in homage to past emperors and thereby venerate them as gods. Pagans of the ancient world found no difficulty in performing this ritual, as they easily accepted the emperor as one of many gods in their polytheistic pantheon. Monotheistic Jews found the ritual abhorrent, but they were excused from making this token political gesture as a consequence of their protected status. Christians, in contrast, were put on trial and punished by death for refusing to conform. For them it was a test of loyalty to the one true God and, as such, a moral challenge of profound importance. To their understanding the consequence of denying Christ was eternal separation from him and banishment to hell. During the ten great persecutions between 61 AD and the official adoption of Christianity as the state religion in 324, several thousand Christians chose torture and death rather than apostasy and damnation.

Like St Peter these martyrs were given the opportunity to deny Christ three times. Pain accompanied each denial. The martyrs' course began the moment they refused to offer the ritual sacrifice. This bold defiance of imperial authority brought them to the attention of the local authority, who arrested them, took them to court and ordered them to recite the oath before a judge. If these Christians refused to comply this second time and instead witnessed to their faith, they were taken to jail, where the state sanctioned torture as a means of persuading the deviants to see the error of their ways and submit. Men and women alike were subjected to the

17

ravages of lions and wild beasts, fire, burning oil and mutilation by sword and club, while women were also threatened with rape. If Christians held fast to their faith and denied the state its due this third time, they faced execution. Citizens died quickly by the sword, slaves slowly on the cross. For both groups heaven was assured along with a hallowed place in Christian history.

No more eloquent paean has ever been composed to the heroism of the martyrs than the testament of St Polycarp, appointed bishop of Smyrna by St John and executed at the age of eighty-six in 155 AD. 'Who would not admire the martyrs' nobility, their courage, their love of the Master?' he began.

> For even when they were torn by whips until the very structures of their bodies were laid bare down to the inner veins and arteries, they endured it, making even the bystanders weep for pity. Some indeed attained to such courage that they would utter not a sound or cry.... Fixing their eyes on the favour of Christ, they despised the tortures of this world, in one hour buying themselves an exemption from the eternal fire.... Similarly did those who were condemned to the beasts endure terrifying torments, being laid out upon trumpet-shells, and bruised by other different kinds of tortures. The purpose was that, if possible, the tyrant might persuade them to deny the faith by constant torment.[1]

The courage displayed by the martyrs from the initial trial to the final swordblow was immense. Contemporaries discovered that it could only be displayed by those whom God called to this particular form of witness and whom he endowed with extraordinary grace to withstand agony and death without flinching. Those who chose martyrdom for their own purposes – self-glorification or peer pressure – generally failed to cope successfully with torture. Their stories were told orally and circulated in writing throughout the Christian communities around the Mediterranean to discourage all but those who believed strongly in their special vocation to martyrdom from putting themselves in danger.[2]

Two valiant female martyrs were Vibia Perpetua, a newly-married twenty-two year old woman who had just given birth to a son, and her pregnant maid, Felicitas. Together they died in 203 AD in North Africa as a consequence of the fifth great persecution. Their plights were not unusual. The uniqueness of their story derives from the fact that Perpetua, herself, recorded their experiences up to the final scene in the amphitheatre. Her writings have become a seminal document in the *Acts of the Martyrs*, a collection of testaments recorded by contemporaries in both Latin and Greek for the encouragement of the faithful.[3] Perpetua's particularly female concerns are heartrending and her chronicle gripping. As soon as she was arrested, her father pleaded with her to renounce her religion to save her baby's life, but Perpetua replied:

> 'I cannot be called anything other than what I am, a Christian.' At this my father was so angered by the word 'Christian' that he moved towards me as though he would pluck my eyes out. A few days later we were lodged in the prison; and I was terrified, as I had never before been in such a dark hole! With the crowd the heat was stifling; then there was the extortion of the soldiers; and to crown all, I was tortured with worry for my baby there. Then [deacons from the local church] bribed the soldiers to allow us to go to a better part of the prison for a few hours. Everyone then left that dungeon and shifted for himself. I nursed my baby, who was faint with hunger.... Then I got permission for my baby to stay with me in prison. At once I recovered my health, relieved as I was of my worry and anxiety over the child....
>
> One day while we were eating breakfast we were suddenly hurried off for a hearing. We arrived at the forum, and straight away the story went about the neighbour-

19

hood near the forum and a huge crowd gathered. We walked up to the prisoner's dock. All the others when questioned admitted their guilt. Then, when it came my turn, my father appeared with my son, dragged me from the step, and said: 'Perform the sacrifice – have pity on your baby!' [Perpetua refused again.] Then Hilarianus [the governor] passed sentence on all of us: we were condemned to the beasts. [Perpetua handed her baby over to a Christian woman.] As God willed, the baby had no further desire for the breast, nor did I suffer any inflammation; and so I was relieved of any anxiety for my child and of any discomfort in my breast.[4]

After recording the visions which she received in chains while still imprisoned, Perpetua ended her commentary. An eyewitness took up the tale through the harrowing final episode. He also told the story of Felicitas, the slavegirl who was eight months pregnant at the time of her arrest and who had not yet given birth by the time of the trial. Roman law forbade the execution of pregnant women out of concern for the paternal rights of the father.[5] Having failed to give birth before the trial, Felicitas was distraught at the prospect of watching her friends go off to the beasts while she was left in the dungeons to give birth and then be executed with common criminals. But two days before the special games arranged to celebrate the emperor's birthday, when her friends were scheduled to provide entertainment for the crowd, she finally had the baby. No sooner had she surrendered the child than she, hand in hand with Perpetua, marched off to the arena. The crowd demanded that they be scourged with metal spikes attached to leather whips before a line of gladiators. The young women were attacked by a mad heifer, while their male companions were mauled by leopards. Perpetua and Felicitas

were stripped naked, placed in nets and thus brought out into the arena. Even the crowd was horrified when they saw that one was a delicate young girl and the other was a woman fresh from childbirth with milk still dripping from her breasts. And so they were brought back again and dressed in unbelted tunics. First the heifer tossed Perpetua and she fell on her back. Then sitting up she pulled down the tunic that was ripped along the side so that it covered her thighs, thinking more of her modesty than of her pain. Next she asked for a pin to fasten her untidy hair: for it was not right that a martyr should die with her hair in disorder, lest she might seem to be mourning in her hour of triumph. Then she got up. And seeing that Felicitas had been crushed to the ground, she went over to her, gave her her hand, and lifted her up. The two stood side by side.... [Perpetua, after exhorting her friends to stand firm in the faith and after being bidden to stand with them in front of the crowd for their final test of loyalty, embraced them in the kiss of peace. Then they all stood silently to await the sword.] Perpetua had yet to taste more pain. She screamed as she was struck on the bone; then she took the trembling hand of the young gladiator and guided it to her throat. It was as though so great a woman ... could not be dispatched unless she herself were willing.[6]

The atrocities visited upon Perpetua and Felicitas and the dignity of their behaviour were mirrored in the lives and deaths of many other women. A literary tradition developed in celebration of their heroism. In some cases historical fact was embellished with inspiring fiction, and in others verifiable biography was abandoned altogether in favour of popular local legend. All of these stories exerted a powerful hold on the Christian imagination.

During the persecution of Marcus Aurelius in which Polycarp perished, for example, it is recorded that a devout woman called Agathonice outraged the proconsul by her un-wavering resolution to elevate her vocation as a Christian above that of wife and mother. The proconsul ordered her to be flung on the pyre where her teachers had just expired. There she died, after shouting her testimony of faith, before the swordsmen arrived to execute her properly.[7] According to North African tradition a beautiful woman called Crispina was doomed to the arena in 304. Fearing that her beauty would elicit the crowd's sympathy, her judge commanded that she 'be completely disfigured by having her hair cut and her head shaved with a razor till she is bald' before entering the arena.[8] Popular hagiographers recorded the tales of Agatha, whose breasts were hacked off,[9] of Faith, who was attached to animals and stretched until she disintegrated,[10] and of Priscia, who was bludgeoned until senseless.[11]

The tortures were ingenious and horrendous. They were meted out to criminals as well as Christians, but the former found few scribes to record their heroism. Perhaps the cruellest torture on record was inflicted in the 280s on Potamiaena, a young woman from Alexandria. Boiling pitch was slowly poured drop by drop over her entire body from her head to her toes. When she survived this without renouncing Christ, she was burned at the stake alongside her mother.[12]

The martyrs perished in excruciating pain. Their example has inspired Christ's followers for nearly two thousand years. The Roman persecutions – dramatic and well-recorded – were only the first chapter, for the book has many volumes and it is not yet complete. Perhaps its conclusion will be written at the end of time just before the second coming of Christ, as the first martyrs predicted. Until then we must recognise the pain endured by the countless numbers of men and women who have died for their faith. In the twentieth century alone millions were killed at the instigation of Stalin in Russia. All were condemned as enemies of the state, yet many were Christians defending their outlawed faith. In Germany some like Bonhoeffer were executed in Nazi concentration camps.

Priests and nuns are still being slain as traitors in South

and Central America, and missionaries are still being slaughtered as imperialist agents in Africa. Throughout this century thousands of Christian nurses, doctors, teachers and aid workers have risked their lives working in mission hospitals, schools and development projects, and hundreds have died while doing so. Their corporate epitaph must be the words of revelation written by St John on Patmos as the first persecutions devastated the tiny Christian community around the Mediterranean:

> I looked and saw a vast throng, which no one could count, from all races and tribes, nations and languages, standing before the throne and the Lamb. They were robed in white and had palm branches in their hands, and they shouted aloud: 'Victory to our God who sits on the throne, and to the Lamb!'...One of the elders turned to me and asked, 'Who are these all robed in white, and where do they come from?' I answered, 'My lord, it is you who know.' He said to me, 'They are those who have passed through the great ordeal; they have washed their robes and made them white in the blood of the Lamb. That is why they stand before the throne of God and worship him day and night in his temple; and he who sits on the throne will protect them with his presence. Never again shall they feel hunger or thirst; never again shall the sun beat on them or any scorching heat, because the Lamb who is at the centre of the throne will be their shepherd and will guide them to springs of the water of life; and God will wipe every tear from their eyes.'[13]

To this confident prediction those of us who live in more peaceful times and countries can only respond 'amen'.

The pain endured by us and by all of the saints whose struggles are recounted in this book differ generically from that of the martyrs. Ours is a force of nature, not of man's inhumanity to man. It is less public, less transparently and immediately Christlike. But it is potentially no less heroic and no less redeeming. The noble army of martyrs is small, but all Christians through the ages have been called to be saints – witnesses of Christ's kingdom on earth – and pain has often been an integral part of that witness.

Chapter Three

The Route of False Martyrdom

THE MARTYRS demonstrated the grace of witnessing to Christ in and through pain, but there is another form of martyrdom available to those in chronic pain. It is false. Almost inevitably melodramatic, it presents a most unedifying spectacle. It is, however, a great temptation, one to which I routinely succumb. As a consequence, I can testify to its potent allure and its devastating effect on others.

False martyrdom is exhibited in the 'poor little me' syndrome. It rests on the assumption that you are heroically carrying on through extreme difficulties, against insurmountable odds. No one is giving you any credit for this herculean achievement – much less trying to make it any easier! The drama is clear. So is the guilt trip on which it sends the entire family, close friends and anyone else who might be deigned to be unaware, unhelpful and unappreciative. The 'victim' of this noble plight struggles on, wounded yet courageous, singing 'he who would valiant be' and alienating everyone he or she meets along the way.

Perhaps the worst travesty of false martyrdom is that your identity as a person is reduced to your suffering. You present your pain as the first – and occasionally the only – obvious point of contact with others. Whereas withstanding staggering pain as a witness to his or her faith is the true martyr's greatest distinction as a person, and the gory instrument of martyrdom is his or her personal symbol, there is far more than pain to distinguish you as an individual. Suffering is a part of your being, and to a degree it contributes to the formation of your personality over time. It is not, however, your whole identity. Asking other people to relate to you primarily through your pain is to close off the rest of your being and reduce yourself to a figure of pathos. It is a huge mistake and a colossal personal tragedy.

The main error of false martyrdom is its presumption that whenever you are in pain you should be able to expect others instantly to recognise your discomfort and practical limitations and accommodate their lives to them. This is a gross form of selfishness. It asks other people to bear burdens which are not theirs and which they cannot possibly carry. Demanding constant attention and assistance turns the person in pain into a tyrannical invalid and those around him or her into slaves.

Few people in chronic pain are false martyrs all the time. The scene is usually set in periods of overwork and stress when everyone at home and work is fraught and the normal give-and-take of relationships weakens under the pressure of more work and less sleep. My greatest annual performance of false martyrdom invariably occurs at Christmas. Every year I vow that I will avoid this star role by buying presents as I see them throughout the year, purchasing cards in September, writing them in October, wrapping gifts in November and enjoying a holy and relaxed Advent. Never have I achieved this idyll. Like every other woman in the Western world, I am exhausted during this festal season. Yet like all others in chronic pain, I am even more drained of good sleep, good will and good cheer. Extra chores deplete the energy I need to stay on top of pain. Shopping, carrying heavy parcels, bending up and down to decorate the tree and house, cooking special treats and entertaining guests make serious demands on waning physical and emotional reserves. Christmas means more pain and less rest, more work and less time to recuperate, more people in the house and less time and space alone for recovery.

Holiday obligations create many more opportunities to feel

pummelled by an impossible schedule, misunderstood by my nearest and dearest, and many temptations simply to blow my top, respond acerbically or simply weep with fatigue and pain. Over the years I have learned the wisdom of limiting direct confrontations by biting my tongue before making a caustic remark. Nevertheless, I can be found at least once over the Christmas holidays retreating to the bathroom, turning on the taps and crying unabashedly. I shall never forget the Christmas day ten years ago when I could not wait to explode and rushed home after the morning service to weep in the nearest private place, which happened to be the coat cupboard. I had just about collected myself when someone opened the door to hang up a child's jacket and found me daubing my eyes and frantically searching in my handbag for powder to cover the red blotches on my face. Summer holidays in a house filled with guests have presented many of the same pressures and identical temptations to false martyrdom. It has taken years to discover how to resist them.

There is a good way to avoid the feeling of too much work, too much pain and too little understanding from others, which provoke you to become a martyr. This is to let others know when you simply cannot respond to them or participate in an activity with them. Several years ago my husband devised a simple 'blue alert' and 'red alert' system which works on those rare occasions when my pride allows me to admit my impending lurch into a situation which I cannot handle. When I whisper 'blue alert' to him it means that I am nearing the end of my tether and that we must complete whatever we are doing in a fairly short period of time. In an art museum this means that I must take a tea break; on shopping expeditions it means we must reduce the list of errands; and when entertaining it means that he must carry a tray upstairs or help serve dinner.

'Red alert' means that I have reached the end of my physical and emotional resources and cannot proceed further. It calls for drastic action. It is generally avoided by 'blue alert', but pride often tempts me to keep going without mentioning decreasing stamina and mounting pain until I have become brittle and bad-tempered. By then a graceful retreat is impossible and withdrawal from the activity is the only way to avoid a provocatively whining remark leading almost inevitably to a row.

The system of coloured alerts is admirable insofar as it allows me to keep my dignity but communicate necessary information. A lovely and gracious friend of my mother achieved the same end by announcing cheerfully that 'Arthur' (her arthritis) was 'visiting' and being ever so demanding whenever she was *in extremis*. This phrase told her friends in the nicest, least guilt-imputing way that her energy and mobility were limited.

I heartily recommend finding a similarly coded way to communicate with your family and close friends so that you obtain the solace of sharing your problems on the occasions when you truly cannot cope with them, and so that those around you become aware of the fact that you are in a particularly bad way and need their understanding and help. But don't do it too often or you will turn this system into an instrument of torture and queue up once again for false martyrdom!

Chapter Four

The Holy Highway:
The Way of Religious

FOR CHRISTIANS of all ages the way of the cross has been the highway to heaven. Relatively few have actually carried a cross or been martyred, but millions have pursued a lifestyle which has kept their eyes keenly trained on the cross as the best means of finding their Saviour. For some the call to 'take up your cross and follow me' has led to a lifetime of self-imposed suffering. Abandoning human society, they have walked an isolated *via crucis* (way of the cross) which has also been a *via dolorosa* (way of sorrow). They have pruned their needs to the barest necessities, exposing themselves to the elements without and the terrors within which seize people when they divorce themselves from humanity.

Single-minded zeal for God's companionship has been rare, for the physical and emotional suffering imposed by such a life demands a special vocation and tremendous stamina. This radical austerity has been embraced by anchorites like St Simon Stylites who lived atop a six and a half foot pillar in Antioch in the fifth century AD, and recluses like St Seraphim of Sarov who built an isolated hut on the Russian steppes in the nineteenth century. In medieval England St Julian of Norwich spent the last years of her life enclosed in a cell attached to a church wall, and in Oxford today one of the older members of the All Saints Sisters of the Poor lives in silence within the convent. Some anchorites and recluses have voluntarily borne hunger and the ravages of climate; all have embraced the rigour of absolute solitude and totally riveted their attention heavenwards. Their prolonged suffering has been as great as any martyr's.

Less obvious and dramatic suffering has been embraced by monks and nuns banding together in community to seek God through corporate prayer and a simple life. Depriving themselves of secular pleasures and creature comforts, they have obeyed a common rule of poverty, chastity and charity, some orders adding stability or obedience as well. Through community rules they have sought to conform their lives to that of Christ.

Among the earliest monastic communities were that founded in Marseilles in the fifth century under John Cassian and that established at Monte Cassino a century later under the great St Benedict. Both monks penned rules for men and women who sought a holy escape from Roman society as the stable imperial regime shattered under the pressure of barbarian invasions. Benedict's rule became a model for the monasteries and convents which proliferated throughout Western Europe from the demise of the Roman Empire to the Reformation of the sixteenth century. It divided the day between agricultural and household work, 'God's work' (the regular recitation of the psalms in choir) and individual rumination on the Scriptures. Its aim was to enable every monk and nun to fulfil St Paul's injunction to 'pray without ceasing'. The life it dictated was basic but not punitively severe. It respected the needs of body, emotions and spirit and imposed a gentle daily rhythm of work, prayer and association through which each of those needs could be satisfied. Insofar as it allowed mortification – killing the lusts of the flesh by fasting and bodily punishment – it cautioned prudence and restraint.[1]

An important goal of the monastic regime was to lead the individual to God through the experience of 'compunction'. This was a very particular kind of suffering. Derived from a Latin medical term referring to acute physical pain, it was adopted by medieval Christians as a theological term referring to spiritual pain. They defined it in two ways. The first was a

painful recognition of one's sinful state and of particular sins
weighing heavily on one's conscience. Experiencing this kind of
compunction, the Christian wept in sorrow for his or her sins.
The second form of compunction was a painful longing for
God's company, an emotional yearning so deep and intense
that it hurt. In this state the Christian wept tears of desire.[2]
Today these terms seem obsolete to many of us in Britain and
North America, for we do not share this vocabulary of religious
experience. However, my South American friends have
retained the word compunction, and they feel no inhibitions in
expressing the deep anguish, sorrow and longing associated
with it. Those of us with stiff Anglo-Saxon upper lips might
profitably learn a wider range of religious experience from
them!

The quest for God produced other forms of pain. These were
admirably described by Thomas à Kempis, a canon who lived
in a priory near Cologne in the fifteenth century. A shrewd
observer of human emotions and behaviour, Thomas à Kempis
appreciated what a struggle it was to find God and live continually in his presence, even in a monastery. His advice
abounds with images of warfare and calls to battle: 'you will
progress in proportion as you do violence to yourself';[3] 'you
must learn to break yourself in many things';[4] 'unless you
apply force to yourself you will not conquer vice';[5] 'you must be
stripped and carry a pure heart to God if you wish to be un-
burdened and to see how sweet the Lord is'.[6] Thomas à Kempis
instructed the individual to denude himself of earthly posses-
sions, attachments and concerns and then to turn his attention
inwards to fight the deadly sins of anger, greed, jealousy, sloth
and selfishness. He assured his readers that the fruits of
victory over self would be humility, patience and peace in this
life and the beatific vision of God in the life to come. Bearing
hurt upon hurt in this life-long battle, the holy warrior would
slowly conquer himself and win the twin trophies of divine love
and eternal rest.

For many religious over the centuries the pains of living in community have been every bit as great as – and often greater than – the pangs of the God quest. An informal survey of friends in several religious orders has yielded insight into this particular kind of suffering. The first is the pain of having one's talents ignored and creativity suppressed. Until quite recently monks and nuns were often seen as interchangeable parts and slotted into jobs without reference to individual interests and expertise. Some now look back in deep sorrow at years of wasted opportunities to benefit their communities and glorify God by developing their unique gifts. For these men and women the collective identity has become increasingly oppressive and painful to bear.

A second kind of pain listed by my friends has arisen from the repression of their emotional lives and the stunting of their emotional growth. Monastic communities are organised like families with fathers or mothers superior. Some superiors have treated their brethren like children, expecting them to be dependent, docile and obedient rather than independent, responsible and emotionally mature.

The third and arguably worst form of pain has resulted from the isolation of the individual in the group. A positive motive for enforced time and space alone has been to ensure scope for the God quest. Another reason has been to prevent so-called 'special friendships' which could threaten the cohesion of the group, as well as overt expressions of sexuality which could lead to scandal. The result of prolonged isolation has been intense loneliness. To live in a group yet to be cut off from it – to be deprived of affection, respect for one's talents and attention to one's particular needs – has turned some monasteries and convents into little outposts of purgatory for those who yearned to bond with their brothers and sisters in Christ and truly live 'in community'.

Today those called to the religious life are facing an all-enveloping pain which is both individual and corporate. It is caused by the need to abandon their familiar, time-honoured ways of witnessing to Christ and to discover radically different ways of incarnating Christian values which are appropriate to the new world emerging at the turn of the twenty-first century. It is a time of trial for religious all over the globe. In the past thirty years their numbers have fallen by one third and their median age has soared to over sixty. Their vitality has been sapped not only by death and departure but – even more demoralising – by a steep fall in the number of youthful aspirants. In the United States, for example, only one per cent of the total religious population is under the age of thirty.[7] Most communities in Western Europe and North America face huge bills for the care of the elderly and the upkeep of large, old and expensive-to-run buildings. Some have gone bankrupt; many have closed. From an outsider's perspective the picture is one of doom and gloom. Yet from within convents and monasteries it is perceived as a time of bereavement mingled with hope and enlivened by a quickly growing sense of liberation.

This odd combination of anxiety and anticipation arises from the capacity of many religious to assess their present situation in an historical perspective. They appreciate that their predecessors have already survived periods of upheaval, apparent death and ultimate reinvigoration.[8] This knowledge gives them courage to persevere and endure their current anguish. The first period of death and rebirth occurred in the early sixth century, when the model of anchorites and hermits withdrawing to the wilderness gave way to a corporate, regulated regime imposed by rules like that of St Benedict. The second occurred in the thirteenth century, when friars and mendicants abandoned cosy, settled monastic enclosures and set out on foot and in utter poverty to preach the gospel in the new towns and cities being built outside feudal strongholds. So popular were the new orders that between the foundation of the Dominicans and Franciscans in the early thirteenth century and the beginning of the Reformation in the early sixteenth century, their numbers rose to roughly ninety thousand.[9]

During the third great upheaval in the history of religious orders, friars, monks and nuns suffered a huge diminution. In the sixteenth century the Protestant reformers took control of England, Scotland, Holland, Scandinavia and many of the German states, closing monastic houses and priories and expelling thousands of men and women to find their way in secular society. The religious life seemed on the verge of collapse, but not for long. The Papacy reacted swiftly by commissioning new apostolic orders like the Jesuits to win back the cultural and social elite of Europe to Roman Catholicism. In the seventeenth century the Holy See sanctioned the foundation of orders for both men and women dedicated to nursing the poor, instructing the uneducated and evangelising Asians, Africans and South Americans.

No sooner had vitality been restored to the religious life by such orders as the Daughters of Charity and the Christian Brothers than the French Revolution of the 1790s sounded yet another apparent death knell, sparking off anticlericalism, the suppression of monastic orders and a full-scale philosophical attack on Christianity itself. Within a few decades the number of religious had shrunk by three quarters and, for the fourth time, the religious life seemed to have reached its end.[10]

In the nineteenth century no fewer than six hundred new communities were founded.[11] Thousands responded to the call to witness to Christ by embracing lives of poverty, chastity and obedience and by evangelising the masses at home and in colonial outposts through work in church hospitals, schools and orphanages. By the Second Vatican Council in 1962 the religious population within the Roman Catholic Church had reached its historical zenith with over two hundred thousand men and women in the United States alone.[12] Dramatically, within less than a decade one quarter renounced their vows, left the religious life and inaugurated the fifth great period of revolution in the religious life.[13]

It is within the context of this corporate historical experience that the present agony of death and rebirth must be viewed. The old monolithic teaching and nursing orders in which brothers and sisters were seen as interchangeable parts embodying the corporate ethos are all but gone. Instead, monks and nuns are increasingly seeing themselves, and being seen by outsiders, as individuals offering particular gifts to their communities and to the groups to whom these communities minister.[14] In many communities the old pattern of absolute obedience to those in authority has given way to group discussions and collegiate decisions. The old theology of transcendence, by which the cloister provided a place apart from the world where men and women could transcend the world in anticipation of heaven, has given way to a theology of incarnation, by which religious men and women live in the world where they strive to embody the heavenly virtues and transform the world on the heavenly model. In some communities long hours of corporate prayer have given way to a more individualised pursuit of the spiritual life. Crucially, the overriding sense of uniform congregational purpose which bound communities together has been largely lost.

Religious are only slowly discovering new visions of how they can witness to Christ in novel ways which make sense in the so-called 'postmodern' world. A recent gathering of distinguished religious defined attributes of their communities in the new age to come:

1. they will live with less;
2. they will be at heart contemplatives basing their endeavours on a rigorous prayer life;
3. they will be prophets criticising social institutions and championing the marginalised;
4. they will invest their time and talents directly in serving the poor, and they will minister where others in the Church and State cannot or will not go;
5. they will embrace a commitment to ecumenism and to other faiths searching for God;
6. they will serve as mediators among the various cultures which make up modern society.[15]

For the moment virtually every community lives in turmoil as the financial and practical pressures of the dying order weigh heavily alongside the challenge to embrace radically different ways of thinking, praying, living and ministering. Each community must go through its own crucible. The only certainty is that those which survive will bear little resemblance to the patterns of witness established in the nineteenth century and sustained into the 1990s.

For our purposes an important observation to be drawn from the experience of religious over nearly fifteen hundred years is that they have embraced a life of prayer and austerity because they have felt called by God to do so. It has quite literally been their vocation, or particular calling. They have answered this call in the full knowledge that they would court compunction and encounter social pain (for want of a better term) by living in communities. But many have also been caught up in waves of historical change which they could not have predicted and which have added an extra measure of suffering. Some have found this new burden more than they could bear and have left their communities. Those who have remained have often felt caught in an excruciating nexus of private and public pain, one which has seemed to have no end. Perhaps unexpectedly, those in chronic pain have much to learn from the sufferings of contemporary monks and nuns.

Chapter Five

Travelling Tips from Monks and Nuns

THE LESSONS offered by religious to those of us in chronic pain are numerous and important. The first is the challenge to incorporate suffering into our vocation as Christians. Monks and nuns are called to follow Christ in an obvious and clearly defined way, but they do not have an exclusive claim to vocation. God calls all of us to respond to him by following Christ. He then challenges us to express our vocations by shaping our identities according to what we discover about him, his kingdom and its values. Monks and nuns have traditionally accomplished this by donning habits and living in community. Those of us in chronic pain do so by using our suffering as one means – and often a very significant one – to develop and define our identities as Christians in the unique circumstances of our individual lives.

The second lesson which we learn from contemporary religious is how to make positive use of deprivation. To pursue their vocations monks and nuns give up personal property, sexual relations and the right to dictate their own affairs. Having surrendered their freedom in all things great and small, they are able to witness to Christ by conforming to the rules of their communities and the dictates of their superiors.

Those of us in chronic pain also surrender our freedom and self-determination to the extent that our suffering intrudes on everyday activities and ultimately on life choices as well, if the suffering is sufficiently prolonged and debilitating. When mobility is severely restricted or long stints in bed are necessary, the deprivation is enormous. When movement is impeded but not halted, or when work and play are circumscribed but not stopped, the deprivations are less dramatic but no less real, especially if they are imposed over many years.

Finally, like monks and nuns, those of us in chronic pain surrender the delusion that we are masters of our own fates on an intimate, daily basis. Conforming to the rules of our doctors and the variable dictates of our conditions, we must weave episodes of deprivation into the pattern of our Christian witness.

It is in answering the question of how to employ pain in a positive response to God that monks and nuns offer the most important lesson. Discipline is the essence of the religious life, and it is also the foundation of positive suffering. Over fifteen hundred years ago, as we have already observed, St Benedict realised that a sane, scrupulously-observed daily pattern of labour, group prayer, private devotion and community social-ising provided an effective framework in which to find God. Countless religious have found not only their vocation but also true contentment in following his rule. Since all Christians are well advised to devise a daily discipline of work, prayer and recreation adapted to the peculiar circumstances of our lives, the disciplines imposed by chronic pain are merely additions to the universal norm and enhancements of it.

In my experience there are four useful disciplines. The first relates to rhythm. Because pain saps energy, it is necessary to pace ourselves and thereby ensure enough rest and sleep to restore the energy supply. To the extent that we try to ignore our discomfort and live a 'normal' life, this is difficult. There are times when the pressure of responsibilities becomes so great that opportunities to rest disappear and the ability to sleep soundly diminishes substantially. These are precisely the times when pacing ourselves is essential and playing 'normal' is disastrous. On these occasions I, for one, used to display a frenetic overdrive which kept me slogging away at the task in hand well past the point at which sensible limits were not only reached but exceeded.

When I was younger the tyranny of the 'to do' list excited mad feats of overextension. The consequence was always loss of perspective, loss of a sense of humour and mounting tension. Depleted of reserves of both energy and patience, I experienced pain more acutely than I would have done if I had had the sense to stop earlier. This is not only because the strain and consequent pain had become worse, but also because I had become far less resilient in mind and body and therefore far less able to cope with any pain at all, let alone a larger dose of it.

Middle age has enabled me to discover that I am not in control of all that once inspired me to these ludicrous exercises in overextension. It has also deprived me of the memory for long lists of obligations. Sweet relief! The consequence is that I no longer feel responsible for everybody and everything in the house, and I no longer feel driven to undertake the demented labours of my youth. Over the years I have also recognised the need to impose periods of rest on my schedule. I nap after lunch on weekends and holidays, I relax on Sundays and I disappear regularly to the convent for weekends of quiet and restoration. Treating myself to more rest, I enjoy more energy and tolerate ordinary pain with little difficulty.

The second discipline relates to maintaining one's body in as fit a condition as possible. St Benedict provided guides on eating, exercising and sleeping, all of which were based on common sense rules for keeping communities of religious healthy as well as happy. For many years my eating patterns have been dictated by two rules. The first springs from advice I was given when young by a wise orthopaedist who told me to stay thin in order to place as little extra pressure as possible on damaged joints. The second arises from the perceived benefit of eating little and often and keeping the energy supply 'topped up' every three to four hours.

The sage orthopaedist also told me to remain as active as possible for as long as possible. To promote and extend mobility he recommended a modest daily exercise regime.

Sadly, I have been too lazy to sustain a consistent programme of exercise over the years. With the exception of walks in the park with the dog, occasional guilt-ridden bursts of stretching and toning, and lovely summertime swims and walks on the beach, I have often failed to include exercise in my schedule. I have paid the price in a gradual deterioration of joints which might have been retarded if muscles had been stronger and more supportive.

My only real discipline in keeping active has been the ludicrously modest one of continually changing position. It is simple, but it helps. At the office I am like a jack-in-the-box, reading and marking reports on the high wide shelf along the back of my desk (which stands at right angles to the wall) and then sitting to type. At home I alternate standing to cook and sitting to write cheques and shopping lists. At parties I alternate sitting and standing. By bobbing up and down at regular intervals I look a bit crazy, but I nevertheless avoid stiffness, backache and frozen knees.

Fitness is a factor not only of adequate exercise, but also of adequate sleep. Whereas St Benedict insisted that monks and nuns make provision for a reasonable amount of sleep, those of us in chronic pain often find this difficult to obtain. In recent years I have learned how to relax and doze when sleep seems impossible. Equally importantly, I have learned to reckon dozing time as part of the nightly rest quotient and thereby avoid feeling deprived and frustrated by lack of real sleep. Some people can pray as they doze and thus discover hours of extra prayer time, but I am not among them. My mind must be a blank not only to sleep, but also to rest. Years ago I taught myself the extremely useful technique of eradicating all thought, relaxing my facial and ankle muscles, crossing my hands on my chest and nodding off. If worse comes to worst in the middle of the night, I employ this napping technique to ensure a bit of real rest. If the night is punctuated by too many painful interruptions, I pray for grace to remain calm and promise to treat myself gently the next day by eliminating extraneous activities from the schedule.

The third discipline does not relate to St Benedict at all, as it is unique to those who live in daily pain. This is the discipline of pain control. The wise orthopaedist of my youth warned me not to keep 'crashing through the pain barrier'. By this he meant finding a golden mean between the tolerable and the intolerable, desisting from activities causing undue strain and pain but not being frightened by those leading merely to routine discomfort. For all of us 'pain', 'discomfort', 'tolerable' and 'intolerable' are highly subjective terms. What you and I call pain may differ, and what each of us calls pain when we are rested and happy will differ significantly from what we call pain when we are tired and discouraged. Nevertheless, we all know when we are doing something which leads us to cross the threshold from the tolerable to the intolerable.

Knowing when and how to stop unduly painful exertions is part of the discipline. Another part is handling pain relievers sensibly and effectively. On the one hand none of us wants to become addicted to opiates, yet on the other hand we do not wish to wallow in needless pain. If we allow pain to mount too high, it takes more medication to diminish the sensation than if we take less earlier. When younger I used to think it noble to wait until I was *in extremis* to take an analgesic, but now I recognise this as both proud and stupid. Likewise I used to regard a massage as the height of hedonistic luxury, but now I appreciate it as a hugely beneficial, as well as hugely enjoyable, means of relaxing taut muscles and restoring a general sense of wellbeing. Indeed, regular professional massage with acupressure and acupuncture has reduced the overall levels of pain and increased mobility and stamina dramatically.

Obviously, in times of distress extreme measures must be adopted: dislocated knees or pulled ligaments must be bound, a strained back rested, and strong pain killers employed initially. However, the normal daily disciplines entailed in moving about, maintaining a sensible weight and dealing effectively with varying pain levels provide me with an easily sustained means of surviving chronic pain without being excessively distressed by it. The key is to follow your disciplines – whatever they may be – with the tenacity of a religious following the rule of his or her community.

The final discipline is the bedrock of monasticism – prayer. Insofar as those of us in chronic pain are more aware than most people of our physical and emotional limitations, we are also arguably more cognisant of our reliance on grace. Unless we regularly draw on copious quantities of it, we are unable to survive recurring pain without destroying the quality of the day for ourselves and others.

Prayer is the vehicle of grace. To prime its engine regular devotion is required. My efforts vary enormously but at the very least include two essentials. One is an invocation of God upon waking and a prayer for divine companionship and guidance throughout the day ahead. It reminds me that the day is God's and that I am simply a small player on a gargantuan stage. This is infinitely encouraging, especially on days when the first sensation is pain and the first thought is the question of how to get through the next sixteen to eighteen hours.

The second essential is a recitation of the prayer of thanksgiving found in the *Book of Common Prayer* at bedtime.[1] I learned this from Archbishop Ramsey many years ago, and the practice has proved invaluable. By forcing myself to rehearse the day's events, I usually discover that the pleasures far outnumbered the pains and difficulties and that even in the most painful days unsuspected pleasures lurked. The recitation of this prayer also obliges me to put each day's experiences in the context of eternity and to raise my eyes above the day's parapet of both pain and pleasure.

Over the years I have discovered several useful aids to daily prayer. One is a small loose-leaf notebook divided into sections for favourite psalms, hymns, prayers and bits of the Bible as well as for lists of intercessions. These choices enable me to enjoy variety of worship while ensuring that I cover the general categories of daily prayer used by Christians over the centuries.

Another device is a gift from one of the friends to whom this book is dedicated – a watch with a countdown alarm. Before meditating, I set it for fifteen, twenty, thirty minutes or whatever is possible, and then I lose all track of time. This watch has a doze button which I can press and after which I can enjoy an additional five minutes without utterly losing my concentration. A non-ticking alarm clock with a snooze button could be used in the same way.

A third device is a three by five inch index card on which I record a quotation or thought which I wish to ponder through the day and which I then tuck into my handbag for ready access. The lines may be from a hymn, the Bible, a poem, a work of fiction or nonfiction. I discovered this simple tool in a biography of Eleanor Roosevelt, and over the years I have found it a huge boon to rumination of the sort advised by St Benedict (rather like a cow chewing its cud, going over the same material again and again throughout the day, slowly savouring and finally digesting it).

All of these are simple devices aimed at strengthening the foundation of prayer in very concrete ways. They are not glamorous but they are effective if employed regularly. As Thomas à Kempis observed, 'habit is overcome by habit',[2] and the habit of prayer is essential to those who hope to practise the art of creative suffering.

Alas, discipline has rather a bad press these days. Nearly a century after Queen Victoria's death we are still over-reacting as a society to the Victorian dedication to duty and discipline. Further, many who came of age in the 1960s and 1970s adopted the agenda of the counterculture to live spontaneously and enjoy immediate self-gratification. In this context those who have entered religious orders to pursue an obvious life of discipline have looked increasingly odd. Throughout Western society we seem collectively to have forgotten the adage that 'genius is ten per cent inspiration and ninety per cent perspiration'. As a consequence, we have ignored the fact that discipline is essential to creation. The only area of modern life in which this truth is firmly grasped is athletics, where the watchword is 'no pain, no gain'. St Paul, the martyrs, Thomas à Kempis and religious through the ages could easily have understood this aphorism. The disciplines of the Christian life are neither numerous nor onerous. They are, however, absolutely essential. Without them we cannot build the new Jerusalem with our creaturely minds and frail bodies.

Chapter Six

The Path that Leads to a Dead End:
The Way of the Dualists and Those Who
Deny the Reality of Pain

DUALISM – dividing life into good and evil – is a beguilingly attractive but dysfunctional way of dealing with pain. It is a path which leads to a dead end. Quite simply and neatly it denies the reality of physical suffering. It posits that a good God could not allow the presence of evil in creation and could not allow his creatures to suffer. Those who have embraced this line of argument have absolved God altogether from responsibility for evil, pain and death. They have postulated a universe in which spirit (created by him) and matter (created by Satan) are forever separate and forever opposed.

Dualists have consigned pain to Satan's world of matter and thus totally outside the scope of God's domain. They have also denied the Incarnation and the belief that Jesus was fully human and fully divine. Instead, they have asserted that he remained exclusively pure spirit, unencumbered by the body and thus unaffected by suffering. In so doing they have cast his pain, and by extension ours too, as evil and utterly irrelevant to the pursuit of wholeness, holiness and redemption.

Over the past two thousand years dualism has attracted millions of supporters. A notable early prophet of this popular heresy was a Parthian called Mani, allegedly born on 14 July 216 in Mesopotamia on the outer frontier of the Roman Empire.[1] Steeped in Zoroastrianism, Buddhism and Babylonian mythology, Mani grafted the story of Jesus onto ancient dualist epics celebrating an eternal battle between God and matter. He proclaimed that Adam was a product of this struggle, possessing an immortal soul of light trapped in a mortal body. He asserted that Adam was liberated by Jesus, a pure spirit sent by God to assure the human race of its heavenly destiny.[2] Mani promised his followers that they could follow the redeemed Adam out of the bondage of matter into the realm of pure light. In preparation for this journey he instructed them to deny all temptations of the flesh, abstain from meat and marriage, undertake lengthy fasts and spend long hours in solitary prayer.[3]

Given this daunting list of obligations, you might reasonably guess that Mani's sect was a distinctly minority taste. Not at all! In his lifetime it spread throughout the Roman Empire and the Indian subcontinent, and it survived in Chinese Turkestan for more than twelve hundred years.[4] Perhaps even more surprisingly, the sect attracted men and women of great intellect and high social position. His most famous convert was St Augustine of Hippo, a self-professed 'Manichean' for nine years before his conversion to orthodox Christianity in 387.

Augustine denounced Manicheanism, and successive ecumenical Church councils sought to eradicate it, but they succeeded in stifling rather than suppressing it. In the tenth century dualism once again emerged as a full-blown heretical movement in the Balkans. A Bulgarian priest called Bogomile inspired his followers to follow Christ, the true spirit, by embracing a life of prayer, chastity and poverty as the only way to escape the prince of darkness and his dungeon of matter.[5] In the twelfth century this movement gathered momentum in Germany, where its followers were called Cathari ('the pure').

By the thirteenth century dualism had attracted so many adherents in France (where its followers were called Albigensians, after Albi, their first urban stronghold) that it rivalled the official church hierarchy. At a time when Roman Catholic priests were widely criticised for moral laxity, the appeal of Albigensianism was great. Seeking the liberation of spirit from body, these dualists advocated an almost ludicrously ascetical life. The leaders, called 'perfecti', refused to touch food, drink or their own bodies and relied on the faithful to feed and bathe them and attend to their most basic bodily functions. The absolute triumph of spirit over matter was their only concern. Illness was inconsequential and suffering meaningless. The attraction of such rugged austerity was magnetic.

The loss of much territory and thousands of souls to the heretics prompted Pope Innocent III to launch a three-pronged attack. In 1215 he commissioned the new order of itinerant Dominican friars to travel throughout the besieged towns and villages and preach orthodoxy to the rebels. He then sanctioned a crusade under Simon de Montfort to slaughter the movement's leaders and destroy its major citadels.[6] At the end of this exceptionally devastating crusade Gregory IX ordered the Inquisition to offer conformity or death to survivors who persisted in heresy.[7] The Pope's draconian measures were successful, and the Albigensian heresy lost its popular appeal. By the end of the fourteenth century it had been eradicated from Europe.

Five hundred years later dualism sprang up again in – of all places – New England. Its source was the mind-cure movement, which had recently swept across Europe as an alternative to traditional medicine. In 1838 Charles Poyen, a French hypnotist, toured New England disseminating the ideas of Franz Mesmer, the Austrian physician who treated his patients through hypnotism. Mesmer, like the ancient astrologers whom he so avidly read, believed that the human mind was influenced by the stars. He asserted that by laying his hands on his patient's head and fixing his eye on the patient's gaze, he could direct a beneficent astral force into the ailing man or woman, restoring harmony with the universe and with it physical health.[8] He called this healing force 'animal magnetism' and employed it with considerable success in treating hysterical conditions.[9]

Charles Poyen found an enthusiastic audience for mesmerism in New England. In *The Bostonians* Henry James celebrated this mania in the comic figure of Dr Tarrant, a 'mesmeric healer' who laid his hands on the heads of infirm old ladies in stylish Back Bay, announcing that 'the mind rules the body with the sceptre of reason' and requiring them to repeat 'I am a child of reason and as such, pure, perfect and without flaw' to regain health.[10] There were many like him, some fraudulent quacks, some sincere. In the twentieth century Norman Vincent Peale's 'power of positive thinking' and Emile Coué's chant 'every day in every way I am getting better and better' programme similar affirmations.

For our purposes the most important figure in the mind-cure movement was Phineas Parkhurst Quimby, an un-tutored scientist–cum–physician from Belfast, Maine. Quimby was a follower of Poyen, and his most famous disciple was Mary Baker Eddy, the founder of Christian Science, a religious sect which became even more strenuous in its denial of the reality of suffering than Mani, Bogomile and the Albigensians.

Mary Baker sought the help of 'Dr' Quimby in 1862 to relieve a variety of nervous complaints she had suffered since childhood.[11] During attacks she sometimes became un-conscious and at other times rigid; sometimes she suffered convulsions; occasionally she hit her head or back as she writhed.[12] Most doctors called to attend upon her diagnosed her 'fits' as hysterical in origin. Several labelled her condition neurasthenia, a popular generic term for female psychogenic maladies. To the mind of the nineteenth century male medical establishment neurasthenia was caused by too much thought for women's small brains to sustain, too much bore-dom for the idle upper and middle classes to tolerate and too many tight, heavy clothes for fashion-conscious females to endure.[13]

Whatever the cause, Mary Baker's attacks persisted. According to her detractors, they were alleviated only by morphine or by rocking in a cradle or swing.[14] In 1843, at the age of twenty-two, she married a successful businessman called George Washington Glover, but within a year she became a mother, a widow and a confirmed invalid.[15] In 1853 she remarried, but this marriage soon ended in divorce.[16] Isolated, penniless and desperate, she received a circular advertising the miraculous cures of Dr Quimby.

Quimby offered what he called 'the science of health'. It was based on the proposition that the patient's faith in a remedy determined the outcome of a treatment. Today, we would call this the placebo effect. Quimby learned the merits of hypnotism from Charles Poyen when Mesmer's disciple visited Maine during his lecture tour of 1838, and he began treating patients with a combination of mesmerism and homeopathy.[17] Gradually, however, he deduced that both were unnecessary. In his observation the curative process was entirely mental, induced by establishing a good rapport with the patient and by using the power of suggestion alone to direct the body's cure.[18] Significantly, he posited that a good God would not – and indeed could not – allow suffering. Instead, he postulated that man brings this on himself by false ideas instilled in childhood and perpetuated in an ever more crippling fashion into adulthood.[19] In Quimby's 'science' we find dualism in its purest and simplest form. Mind and body are totally separate, and the former is superior because of its relation to the divine. Address the mind, he asserted, and you will treat the disease.

Mary Baker Eddy (as she became in 1877, when she married her third husband, Asa Gilbert Eddy) developed Quimby's ideas into a system which she popularised as 'Christian Science'. Whereas Quimby and his mesmerising friends had asserted the triumph of mind over matter, Mrs Eddy denied the reality of matter altogether. For her the only reality was God, the 'Divine Mind'. Whatever could be adduced by the five senses was not 'of the Mind', and therefore was not real. Obesity, for example, was not a physical state, rather 'an adipose belief of yourself as a substance'.[20] Food was unnecessary. 'We have no evidence', she asserted, 'of food sustaining

Life, except false evidence.'[21] Sickness could only be cured by treating the spiritual ailment.[22] In combatting fever she advised the patient to recognise that heat and chills were 'nothing but an effect produced upon the body by images of disease before the spiritual sense . . ., the effect of fright'. Her remedy was to eliminate the image, vanquish the fright and thus destroy the disease.[23]

Not only recovery from mortal ills, but also the attainment of life immortal was contingent upon correct analysis of the human predicament and correct thought. Mrs Eddy believed that humanity could avert both sickness and death by acquiring the mind of Christ, the greatest 'scientist' of all time. This heightened level of spiritual awareness bestowed the power to heal oneself as well as others and to be healed forever.[24]

The arch-demon in Mrs Eddy's cosmology was Mesmer's 'animal magnetism'. While Mesmer and Quimby had regarded this as a power for good, Mrs Eddy identified a potential for evil, labelling this destructive force 'malicious animal magnetism'. Through it she believed that people could assault their enemies with disease and death. When confronted by recurring bouts of illness, Mrs Eddy ascribed their origin to evil thoughts emanating from former, disgruntled pupils. 'Now Dr Spofford,' she addressed one such renegade,

> 'won't you exercise reason and let me live or will you kill me? Your mind is just what has brought on my relapse and I shall never recover if you do not govern yourself and turn your thoughts wholly away from me. . . . It is mesmerism that I feel is killing me it is mortal mind that only can make me suffer. [*sic*] Now stop thinking of me or you will cut me off soon from the face of the earth.'[25]

When her husband collapsed in 1893, Mrs Eddy ignored the diagnosis of heart disease made by a doctor whom she summoned in desperation and instead insisted that 'it was poison that killed him, not material poison, but mesmeric poison'. As she approached her own death, Mrs Eddy remained convinced that her ailments were the assaults of malicious animal magnetism sent by malevolent former pupils who wished to destroy her and her now very successful movement, which included a huge 'Mother Church' in downtown Boston, a publishing house, a distinguished national newspaper, reading rooms throughout the country and the support of one per cent of the American people. Ordering a twenty-four hour watch of faithful followers to sit outside her bedroom door, she exhorted them to ward off the venomous attacks.[26] Despite their valiant fight, 'Mother' (as she was known to her many followers) 'passed on' in her ninetieth year. Likened to Jesus in sharing the 'Divine Mind', she was hailed by Christian Scientists as the greatest disciple since St Paul.

The popularity of Christian Science has waned since World War Two, but in recent years it has attracted much publicity as a consequence of several court cases in which Christian Scientist parents have been indicted for child abuse and manslaughter. Firmly believing that orthodox medicine is useless in fighting the assaults of malicious animal magnetism, they have refused their children medical care for cancer, appendicitis and a variety of treatable, but otherwise terminal, diseases. Dismissing life-threatening illness as nothing more than a mistaken idea, they have watched their children die rather than admit the reality of matter. 'We finally have come to the point where you place God before your own life,' one mother observed as her twelve-year-old daughter lay dying with an agonising forty-one inch tumour distending her right leg.[27]

In most American states Christian Scientists have won immunity from prosecution through an appeal to the constitutional right to religious freedom and the corollary right to rely on spiritual treatment through a recognised Church rather than physical treatment through the medical profession. However, in the few states which have not granted immunity, they have been tried and convicted of felonies for failure to take the appropriate steps to save their children's lives.[28]

The plight of dying Christian Scientist children is immensely sad, but so, too, is the situation of all those who pursue the pathway of dualism. They devise maps charting a straight spiritual route to heaven by circumventing illness and death. The orthodox Christian route is far less clear, far muddier, far harder to read and far tougher to tread, but it covers the entire terrain of human existence. It bids us follow the example of God's son and endure suffering with our eyes open, our bodies hurting and our emotions fraying. It promises the companionship of the Holy Spirit, who dispenses grace, strength and comfort along the way. It asks us to recognise that we mortals are not omniscient, that we do not know and cannot be certain of the details of humankind's destiny. It challenges us to grow in understanding by living with the tension between doubt and faith. It quite simply asks us to accept – even in this technological age – that human life is ultimately shrouded in mystery.

Because it eschews an entirely rational approach to life, the Christian path is more difficult to describe than routes which supply logical solutions to life's basic problems. This has recently been made very clear to me when, in the course of a month, my husband's thirteen-year-old godson was confirmed and his father killed in an accident. Both he and my fourteen-year-old son have demanded unambiguous responses to straight questions. Are prayers answered? Is there life after death?

I cannot supply black and white answers. I can only respond in the colours of experience. Prayers are answered, yet often in ways we do not expect or readily perceive. Life is a journey which stretches from here into eternity: God does not define the entire route and does not offer a brochure of the final destination, but he does accompany us on the journey and provide grace as fuel to pursue it to its fulfilment. The Christian pathway through life must be tried and tested rather than proved or disproved. As a Christian, I cannot explain life and death to the boys, but I can encourage them to weave faith and hope into their encounters with pain and death. It is my sacred duty to inspire them to step forward into what I believe to be the path that leads to the fullest and noblest life possible.

Chapter Seven

The Challenging Path of Detachment

NONE OF US can avoid asking the fundamental questions posed in the last chapter, for pain is inextricable from the human condition. Our answers are of paramount importance. They determine not only our path through pain, but also the direction of our journey through life itself. What, we ask, is the relationship between God and our pain? Is he in any sense responsible for it? If so, is he a deity whom we can trust? If we trust him, what impact does this have on our suffering?

As we have begun to appreciate, there are several approaches to these questions. Two are beguilingly logical but unsatisfactory to my understanding. One is the atheist's response: that a good God could not create a universe filled with so much suffering. As pain clearly abounds, God cannot exist. The second answer – that of the dualists – starts from the same premise, but instead of denying the existence of God, it denies the existence of pain. God remains good and the problem of suffering is simply eliminated. Neither of these approaches actually helps people in pain. Both require that they divorce their minds from their bodies, satisfying the one but ignoring the other. This severing of explanation from experience surely creates a tension which increases the existential pain and intensifies the suffering.

There is a third approach, one which is less tidy but which unites mind and body and which acknowledges the uncertainties of human life more honestly as well as more hopefully. It is the belief that God is good and wills good for all of us, yet he allows evil to exist. If he is omnipotent and omniscient – and I believe that he is both – he is as responsible for creating the potential for evil as the potential for good. But this is not the end of the story: it is only the beginning. God participates in the cosmic act of redemption. Through the Incarnation he thrust himself into the miseries and agonies of human existence. Jesus, true man and true God, suffered and died in order that suffering humanity might be made forever whole. Through the Holy Spirit, God participates in the struggle of the universe as it agonisingly evolves into a new creation. He also joins with each of us, while we explore the potential for good and wholeness amidst crippling, life-denying pain.

In other words, God gets his hands dirty with the blood, toil, tears and sweat of human suffering. He doesn't give us a neat answer to the problem of pain, but he does give us a way to cope with it and an ultimate meaning to it. He stands as the fount of all goodness at the beginning of creation, at the end of time and on the outer bounds of the universe. Yet he also walks with us through the mess and distress of our mortal lives, offering a vision of ultimate truth, beauty, peace and love. The challenge for us is to train our sights on him as both the fulfilment of life and as the means of reaching that fulfilment. So far as I can ascertain, this is the only means of enduring the evil while trusting in the good, thereby surviving the pain.

If you subscribe to this answer to the problem of pain, the real question becomes: how can you keep your eyes fixed on God? There are so many attractions in the world outside and so much turmoil in our inner emotional lives which obstruct that clear view. Our apparent 'mission impossible' is to detach ourselves from these gigantic obstacles. In practical terms this means prizing ourselves loose from everything that impels us to make ourselves the centres of our universe rather than God. It demands that we resist being controlled exclusively by our own selfish wants, needs and desires and that we desist from trying to control those around us. This willed process of vanquishing our compulsion to satisfy our own egos at all times and in all places as well as to dominate others is not a goal in itself. It is the essential precondition to attaching ourselves to God. It enables us not only to state that God is the centre of the universe, but also to keep a clear eye focused on him day by day. Beneficially, it promotes a peaceful coexistence with our inner emotions and with those around us. It liberates us to enjoy people and things, not possess them. Ultimately, it provides 'perfect freedom' insofar as this is attainable in our earthly lives.

There are several arenas in which detachment can be pursued by all of us, not simply by those of us in pain. The first is human relationships. When I was younger I used to ponder how those of us who live outside convents and monasteries and who enjoy strong and abiding links with family and friends, can detach our affections, and perhaps even more importantly, why we should even try to do so. Jesus' great commandments to love the Lord our God with all our heart and soul and mind and to love our neighbours as ourselves seem to preclude severing the secure bonds of affection. Further, if in the evening of our lives we are to be tried by our love, as St John of the Cross so eloquently predicts, shouldn't those bonds be as tight as humanly possible?

It took years of marriage for me to realise that love which is passionate yet durable exists on three levels, and that detachment is necessary on all of them if the relationship is to remain vital. The foundation is an abiding, profound, unshakeable love – bound for me by the sacrament of marriage – which the fluctuations and frustrations of daily life cannot erode. Detachment on this level occurs when we recognise that love even of this intensity is a gift, as is the companionship of the beloved. This love is fallible and human, contained in time and space. It is bestowed by God, who alone sustains us with a love which abides through time and space.

The second level of deep human love is more concrete and often difficult to handle. It relates to the patterns of daily life, to family plans and career designs, to the rhythm of work and pleasure, to those areas in which I have strong views and a big investment in what my husband and I choose. It is sometimes well-nigh impossible for me to allow him the scope to do as he sees fit without constant reference to my own grand schemes. Despite the enormity of the challenge, I appreciate the need to detach myself as much as possible and afford him the freedom to evolve in ways which I could never imagine and which I as a wife stifle at my peril. Detachment in this area is a great discipline.

The third level of human love is the most superficial and the most taxing. It is riveted on the petty decisions of daily life: to have dinner when he wants it, to leave work early for a concert which he wishes to attend and to do myriad other small things which impinge upon my own schedule and preferences. Detachment in these areas does not mean becoming a door-mat. It means recognising that his needs are as compelling as my own, his wishes as legitimate and his choices the ones that should prevail as often as not. None of these often agonising acts of self-surrender would be possible without the supreme abandonment of all that I am – now and into eternity – to God as the ultimate focus of my love and the only recipient of my adoration.

Curiously, I have found it far easier to detach myself from my son than my husband. Perhaps this is because he was born after several miscarriages, and as a result I have always regarded him as pure gift. Perhaps it is also because I had no preconceptions about how we should relate. As an only child and without brothers, I knew nothing about boys' particular needs and behaviour. Unencumbered by the model of my own extremely close relationship with my mother, I lacked a template of experience to impose on our relationship, and as a happy consequence we both have been truly free to enjoy each other. In this sense I have been detached and watched him grow in wonder and pleasure since the day he was born.

In another sense I have learned detachment by sharing my son with other women who have helped care for him during his childhood. Having relinquished any exclusive sense of maternal control over him, I have stood back – at times with a wrenched heart – and watched him confer affection and loyalty on them. In the end my self-restraint has provided him not with mother substitutes, but rather with substitute sisters, aunts and grandmothers, real treasures for a child whose only close relatives are his parents.

If family relationships have provided one arena in which to pursue detachment, life's activities have provided another. Working in a small team amidst a larger organisation has offered daily opportunities to detach my ego from my professional endeavours. I have found this particularly tricky on occasions when I have worked virtually single-handedly or led a team on big projects. Assuming a corporate identity has sometimes been beyond me, and I have choked on my pride! Likewise, detaching my ego from my writing has frequently seemed impossible. While engaged in the process of writing an article or book I am lost in the creative experience, blissfully unaware of myself and wonderfully cognisant of God's proximity; yet upon the completion of a piece, my ego attaches itself to the finished product like superglue.

Sadly, pride in achievements and emotional megalomania in relationships are not the only, or indeed the most resistant, obstacles to detachment. Routine is far worse. How can we find God at the centre of our lives when so many of our daily activities happen as a matter of habit, without forethought or examination along the way? How can we break into busy schedules and remember that God is at the centre of our small worlds, not we ourselves? We have already been offered practical guidance by the martyrs and religious, and we shall be provided with more by St Teresa of Avila and St Thérèse of Lisieux in the chapters ahead.

For the moment it is vitally important to realise that detachment is not simply a pathway to God, one which is sometimes hard to find and often hard to follow. It is a route which leads to the great highway trodden by all of suffering humanity, who are your companions along the way. To miss this connection is to misread the Christian map and pursue the popular but arid journey of self-fulfilment. If the process of self-detachment and divine attachment does not promote a heightened awareness of others, if it does not open the traveller's eyes to all who struggle with pain and promote a loving concern for them, then it becomes yet another blind alley.

In the modern world 'love' is an overused word with a plethora of meanings. In the ancient Christian context it had two which are highly germane to those of us in pain today. The first is *agape*. Translated as *caritas* by those who produced a Latin Bible from the Greek and 'charity' by those who translated the Bible into English, it means a disinterested but generous regard for our fellow human beings. Today we associate this kind of love more often with voluntary organisations than with a personal disposition of care for others, but they spring from the same thoughtful and giving attitude of mind and heart. Although Christ bade all of his followers to love one another, those of us in chronic pain sometimes find this injunction particularly difficult to heed. Pain at its worst makes us myopic in vision and relentlessly self-centred in consciousness. It blinds us to the wider needs of humanity and produces a debilitating self-preoccupation. A disciplined turning of the gaze outward is in my experience the only way to acquire and maintain a loving concern for people whose sufferings and needs are at least as worthy of attention as my own.

The second definition of love which is deeply meaningful to those in chronic pain is *philia* or brotherly love. This is a closer, more intimate affection for others than *agape*, one akin to family relationships. Because of its greater intensity and intimacy, it is more easily concentrated on individuals than groups. This kind of love enables us to reach out of the depth of our own suffering and empathise with other people in pain. It opens wide the road to compassion, which in Latin literally means 'suffering with'. It identifies those whom you directly encounter in pain as brothers and sisters, and it obliges you to stand beside them, often in prayerful silence, as they grapple with their own suffering. If you lack eyes to see pain of whatever sort in the eyes of those around you, and if you lack the capacity to feel not only for them but with them, you have not detached yourself from your own ego or attached yourself to God. In my experience the call of the Almighty is always outward: away from self towards others, upward towards him and his glory, and forward into eternity, which begins with the present moment.

The ultimate rewards of detachment are liberation and fellowship. Whereas denial and dualism leave us imprisoned in ourselves, detachment frees us from the shackles of self-centredness. It enables us to find meaning in our painful lives by searching for God and discovering the companionship of both the Holy Spirit and of fellow sufferers along the way. It demands honesty, dedication and discipline, but the journey is well worth the effort. It leads to life in its greatest possible abundance both here and into eternity.

Chapter Eight

A Road to Disaster:
The Way of Masochism

A PATHWAY leading to intensified pain – one which has been even more popular than dualism – is masochism. Over the centuries far too many Christians have embraced it in the mistaken notion that they were serving their Lord by punishing themselves. We shall look at two groups in particular. First, we shall study that large group of Christians who have cared for the ill and marginalised in society and lived valiantly generous lives, but who have been driven by a tragic inner emotional poverty. Then we shall examine the fascinating but far smaller group of so-called 'holy anorectics', whose asceticism has led to debility and even death.

At first glance masochism seems an odd diagnosis for a Christian. The Viennese psychiatrist who first coined the term, Richard von Krafft-Ebbing, defined it in his *Psychopathia Sexualis* of 1886 as a perverted means of deriving sexual pleasure. He argued that the masochist obtains erotic satisfaction from submission to the cruel, sadistic behaviour of another. Through a distorted pursuit of sexual excitement the sadist (usually a man) and the masochist (almost invariably a woman) unite in sexual bondage.[1] In his survey of sexual psychopathology Krafft-Ebbing presented sado-masochism as a distinctly minority taste and activity. Its only interest to Christians lay in its generation of sin and misery.

In the years before World War One Freud identified masochism as a far more widespread phenomenon than Krafft-Ebbing's definition would suggest. Indeed, in 1909 he wrote to Jung: 'In my practice, I am chiefly concerned with the

61

problem of repressed sadism [i.e. masochism] in my patients; I regard it as the most frequent cause of the failure of therapy.'[2] Explaining it as a clash between the two instincts of eros (the drive towards pleasure) and thanatos (the death instinct), he raised it to the level of universal experience. He hypothesised that guilt about forbidden sexual impulses is satisfied in the search for punishment through pain.

The sexual expression of this search is limited. Men occasionally display it in the desire to be beaten, to be castrated, to be treated like naughty, helpless children in play or like passive females in sex. Women more frequently exhibit it simply by enduring cruel acts and yielding with pleasure.[3] Sexual masochism as defined by Freud is more frequently a problem for women than men. During the past fifteen years masochism has been radically redefined as a common, persistent and difficult to treat condition. In 1987 masochism was listed in *The Dictionary and Statistical Manual of Mental Disorder III Revised (DSM III–R)*, an international directory of psychiatric terminology, as a self-defeating personality disorder.[4] The specifically sexual basis of masochism has been eliminated. Its origin has now been traced to the lag between physical birth and psychological birth. This begins in the infant's first three years, which are a period of psychological gestation when she experiences herself and her environment almost exclusively in terms of her mother, as she did in the womb during her physical gestation. In the fourth year the toddler and mother must work through a process of separation so that the child becomes an independent individual, one who feels loved and supported but inspired to be herself. This is a normative prescription for mental health. All mothers fail to fulfil it in various degrees, for even the best of us cannot work out the ideal balance between symbiosis and separation in all circumstances. No mother always lets go when she should for her child's optimum emotional development. Her power to impede the child's independence engenders frustration – and even rage. The thwarted child never loses a residual sense of oppression from these experiences.[5]

During this critical learning period the toddler who later develops clinical masochism is particularly oppressed and becomes excessively enraged. Perhaps her mother is too over-burdened with other children or responsibilities to invest enough time and emotional energy to nurture the child properly. Maybe she is too emotionally unstable to offer meaningful support to anyone else. Whatever the reason, she neglects rather than succours. She punishes rather than accepts the child's limitations in comprehension and motor control. She induces guilt in the child for being inadequate from her perspective and, as a consequence, unlovable.

She puts her child into a terrible bind. Rather than risk losing her mother – the worst fate a child can imagine – the child adopts her mother's image of her as her own and accepts responsibility for the failed relationship. But the child is furious with this role reversal and anxious for revenge. Her only means of expressing smouldering rage at being so abused and devalued without jeopardising the relationship is to attack herself through illness, misbehaviour or non-achievement. Through suffering she wins attention of some sort, usually pity, which she confuses with love.[6]

As she grows older, the masochist becomes locked in a pattern of self-defeating activities and relationships in an ongoing, abortive attempt to win affection. She pursues jobs and interests which lead to disappointment rather than achievement and chooses friends who mistreat rather than cherish her. If she happens to succeed in an undertaking or relationship, she feels guilty. If someone offers to help her, she rejects the offer and then feels hurt, defeated and humiliated if that person subsequently rejects her. If opportunities for pleasure arise, she ignores them. If people treat her well, she avoids them. She chooses jobs which are beneath her abilities. She sacrifices herself to work and people when such sacrifices are inappropriate, unsolicited and unwanted. She is depressed much of the time. She need demonstrate only five of these seven characteristics in order to conform to the modern definition of masochism and merit clinical treatment.[7]

The implications for Christianity of masochism in its modern guise are profound and unexplored. Churches, vicarages, convents and monasteries are filled with stereotypically and, indeed, actually good people who also fit the masochistic model. But the disorder is not limited to religious professionals: it can be found in Christian families as well. Indeed, it may be endemic in Christian society. The model of Christian service is the person who gives of himself or herself unstintingly, who perseveres in generosity whatever the obstacles, who is self-sacrificing, self-deprecating and affectionate in the widest sense of the word.

The pathology and tragedy lie not in the attempt to incarnate Jesus's virtues, but rather in the hidden emotional force which drives many to display such nobility of spirit. The mainspring of their activity, unlike that of their Saviour, is an emotional deprivation which few would admit. In childhood they learned to feel valued in caring for others. They also learned to assert control over relationships to ensure that they remain invulnerable to humiliation, hurt and abandonment. Unable to accept the free gift of love from others, they feel compelled to earn love through suffering. Their charity abounds, but so does their pain. Thanked by others, they do not consider their gifts as valuable. Exhausted, they nonetheless keep sacrificing, for they lack the self-respect to set reasonable limits. Loved and admired, they turn away in a desperate attempt to protect themselves from repeating their personal tragedy of infant exposure and rejection. They truly give and do not count the cost.

Because they suffer in silence and outwardly embody the virtues of humility and charity, Christian masochists rarely receive professional attention. Only when depression overwhelms them, or when their self-defeating mechanisms create a crisis, do they seek help. Even then, their chances of recovery are small. Recent clinical surveys prove masochism to be as resistant to treatment today as it was in Freud's time. Antidepressants can ease the pain of low mood, but it takes years of group and individual therapy to heal the psychic wound and engender enough self-worth to adopt new patterns of being, doing and relating.[8] The Church has benefitted from the labours of masochists for centuries. It is now time to recognise the staggering personal cost of masochistic self-sacrifice and extend a compelling, healing love emanating from the divine source.

If courting pain to win love and approval is a common but largely unconscious Christian experience, inflicting pain on oneself to the point of death is nowadays a rare but entirely conscious way to pursue the way of the cross. Recently, a lively controversy has been excited by 'holy anorexia' – women starving themselves to death in pursuit of sanctity. Although most recorded cases of holy anorexia are medieval, the French mystical philosopher Simone Weil is an excellent modern example. A university lecturer, she ate no more than French factory workers' rations during World War Two and she finally starved herself to death in solidarity with those being killed in Nazi concentration camps. The stirring debate on holy anorexia was kicked off by the psychiatrist, Rudolph Bell, and the medieval historian, Caroline Bynum. They question whether medieval women's refusal to eat – sometimes even to the point of death – was basically pathological (Bell) or an expression of healthy female piety (Bynum). To follow their argument we shall examine the causes and symptoms of anorexia nervosa, the modern model for holy anorexia, and the idiom of medieval female spirituality, which diverges dramatically from the more familiar masculine imagery and expression.

Anorexia nervosa was first identified as a disease at least three hundred years ago. It was called anorexia from the Greek *an* meaning deprivation, *orexus* meaning appetite, and *nervosa* meaning psychic rather than somatic in origin. The name is a misnomer insofar as the anorectics never lose their appetite. In fact the most salient feature of the disease is that they fight the urge to eat day in and day out, sometimes to the point of starvation and death. Anorexia nervosa primarily afflicts teenage girls, but in about five per cent of cases males (most famously the poet, Lord Byron) manifest symptoms of the disease.[9] In the 1970s one small-scale British survey of girls aged fourteen to nineteen indicated that four per cent of those studied showed signs of anorexia, and a more ambitious contemporary Scandinavian study estimated a figure closer to ten per cent.[10] Over the last fifteen years clinical studies suggest that the figure has slowly but steadily increased.[11]

In an attempt to treat this stubbornly intractable disease psychiatrists have searched for causes and have discovered contributing factors in family circumstances as well as wider social expectations. They have noted a tendency for the parents of anorectics to be older than the general population as well as middle or upper middle class.[12] They have recorded a high incidence of alcoholism among fathers and psychosomatic disorders such as migraine headaches among mothers.[13] They have raised the possibility of genetic factors, as there is often more than one anorectic in a family.[14] They have observed a family preoccupation with food, faddish diets and physical fitness.[15] Significantly, they have witnessed an extreme family closeness, a resistance to change and an inability to resolve difficulties smoothly.[16] Finally, they have set all of these variables of family circumstance in the context of a society which defines women's fashion and female beauty in terms of thinness. Visitors to Madame Tussaud's London waxwork museum voted for Elizabeth Taylor as the most beautiful woman in the world before 1970, but since then models like Twiggy have usurped this position. Likewise, in the United States the winners of the Miss America contest have consistently weighed less than the average weight of other contestants since 1970.[17] One psychiatrist has called this emphasis on near-emaciation the 'pathology of appearance' and has remarked on the 'democratisation' of anorexia as young women of all social classes have begun to pursue the ideal of exaggerated slimness.[18]

The typical anorectic displays symptoms of the disease before she is twenty-five years old, usually between the ages of fourteen and nineteen. She loses at least one quarter of her body weight. She suffers from no other medical or psychiatric illness which could account for that weight loss. She exhibits a distorted attitude towards food and her own weight. She may engage in bulimic behaviour as well. She may die as a consequence of the disease.[19]

Why does she starve herself, perhaps to death? One persuasive answer is that she is a bright, accommodating teenager who feels trapped by other people's expectations. Seeking to define her individuality, she seizes control of the only thing which is uniquely hers – her own body – and over this she exerts rigid self-control. The more other people criticise her eating habits and despair of her advancing emaciation, the greater the sense of autonomy and achievement. She is no longer a slave to others. Were she to admit that she suffered from an illness and abide by her physician's prescriptions, she would enslave herself once again. To her mind it would be better to die than to surrender.[20]

An alternative explanation is that the anorectic is threatened by the process of maturation, both biological and psychological, and strives to avoid it. Through ruthless dieting she preserves a pre-adolescent figure, and by slimming to the point at which menstruation ceases, the female anorectic reverses puberty. Frightened of rebelling against family values and cohesion like a normal teenager, she fails to negotiate her independence and learn to function separately.[21] Whatever the underlying motive, the result is the same: the anorectic reacts to the threat of growing up by concentrating on her body. She persuades herself that she will feel more in control of her life and better about herself if she loses weight and continues to do so.

According to Bell the holy anorectic bears a remarkable

67

similarity to the modern emaciated teenager. She is an intelligent girl who is notable for her anxiety to please others. At some point during adolescence she rejects their expectations along with society's assumptions about the place of women. Instead, she vows to become holy, as today's young vow to become thin. Grooming herself to become a bride of Christ, she makes herself loathsome to potential human husbands. In her quest to avoid suitors she may disfigure herself through scourging her face, impaling her breasts with metal nails or donning filthy rags.[22]

Seeking to overcome every bodily impulse – hunger, sexual desire, fatigue and pain – she seeks nourishment in the communion wafer alone and deprives herself of sleep. Rapidly, she loses weight. Sexual desire disappears with her periods. She feels exhilarated by her bodily conquests and euphoric in her intimacy with God. For a time she becomes hyperactive despite lack of nourishment, and during this stage she may undertake an impressive array of good works. She feels so ecstatic that no one can persuade her to abandon her course. A perfectionist, she sets no limits to her mortifications. Finally, she collapses through fatigue and malnutrition. Dying, she experiences total liberation from the flesh as she embraces the divine.[23]

The most fully documented illustration of this pattern is St Catherine of Siena, whose biography was a bestseller for two hundred years. Born into a rich mercantile family in 1347, Catherine Benincasa was a highly intelligent, headstrong little girl who showed no early signs of excessive piety. At birth her twin sister died, leaving Catherine as the spoiled surviving infant.[24] When she was two, the plague described by Boccaccio in *The Decameron* hit Italy and the family business foundered.[25]

When Catherine was twelve her beloved older sister died, and when she was sixteen her parents pressed her to marry the grieving brother-in-law, who was rich but considerably older than she.[26] In the same year her younger sister died. Overcome by a sense of guilt at living after her sisters had died and panicking at the prospect of marrying her gauche brother-in-law, she made a bargain with God. In return for the guarantee of salvation for all of her relatives, she would embrace a life of radical piety.[27] As an outward sign of this pact she cut off her long blond hair, put an iron chain around her hips, replaced her fine garments with a crude woollen shift and limited her diet to bread, water and raw vegetables. Flagellation with the chain inflamed her skin and insufficient food reduced her weight by half within months.[28] 'Daughter, I see you already dead,' her mother wailed; 'without a doubt you will kill yourself. Woe is me!'[29] Neither her parents nor her confessors could persuade her to abandon her punishments of the flesh.

Despite her weak state Catherine undertook extraordinary acts of charity as she cared for the sick and dying. In 1376 she went to Avignon to beg Pope Gregory XI, who admired her extreme piety, to return to Rome, take up his proper role and cleanse the Church of lax practices.[30] When Gregory died en route to Rome, she implored his successor, Urban VI, to take up the cause of Church reform. She also attempted to organise a community of women to fast and pray for his success.[31] To advance her own perfection she gave up bread and existed on water and bitter herbs. When her efforts at renewing the papacy and the Church failed, she became despondent, gave up water and died three months later in 1380. She was canonised in 1460.[32]

That Catherine of Siena starved to death is incontestable. Why she did so remains unclear. Her own vocabulary of experience offers a different interpretation of her life and death than one of holy anorexia. As Bynum points out, food was a central image in medieval female piety. Whereas men focused on the dichotomies of wealth versus poverty and sex versus chastity as the essentials of male spirituality, women looked to the homey images of food, gestation, family and suffering for their imagery.[33] In the eucharist they found the perfect sustenance, for the consecrated bread was nothing less than the body of Christ. It was also a communal meal, one which Jesus enjoined on his disciples at the Last Supper and one consumed by the faithful together as the local family of Christ's followers. By limiting her diet to the communion bread, Catherine gave up her own meals for the poor and in so doing followed the law of charity in addition to the dictate of piety.

It is not surprising that Catherine's most famous and numerous miracles were those of feeding. During her lifetime she was attributed with turning sour wheat into sweet and multiplying loaves of bread. After death she was credited with cooking dinner for the family of a woman who had gone to church rather than prepare the evening meal.[34] Her biographer was quick to draw the conclusion that despite the barrenness of her own body she fed and healed others and acted like a mother to all. 'The whole city was in commotion,' he observed. 'Everybody . . . flocked to catch sight of her. "What a woman!" they said. "One who drinks no wine herself, but can by a miracle fill with wine an empty cask!"'[35] Catherine interpreted her aversion to food and her stomach pangs as the pains of purgatory which she suffered on behalf of her family.[36] She firmly believed that by depriving herself and helping others, she was imitating Christ's passion in the most profoundly meaningful way open to any Christian.

The pattern of abstention and charity embraced by Catherine of Siena remains an abiding model of female spirituality. Focusing on the two hundred and sixty-one Italian women canonised between 1200 and 1990, Rudolf Bell and Donald Weinstein calculate that the biographical data are too limited to reach valid conclusions about the eating habits of one third, but that of the remaining one hundred and seventy, at least half exhibited holy anorexia.[37] Less punitively and more commonly generations of pious men and women have followed the habit of refraining from eating before receiving communion. St Teresa of Avila went so far as to induce vomiting by poking the back of her throat with an olive twig to empty her stomach in preparation for the heavenly food.

Whether the aim was purification or charity, abstention was a predominant aspect of women's spirituality until the twentieth century. It has slowly been abandoned as opportunities have arisen for women to work in the slums, hospitals and mission fields and pursue an active life of service rather than the traditional one centred on *Kinder*, *Kirche*, *Küche* (children, church, cooking). To the extent that contemporary female spirituality focuses on influencing the environment rather than controlling the body, it is far healthier than spiritualities motivated by dualism, masochism and holy anorexia.

Chapter Nine

The Pitfalls of Masochism Today

'YOU CANNOT possibly write about masochism,' exclaimed a distinguished criminologist friend of mine upon learning that I intended to tackle this most difficult and taboo of subjects. 'The feminists will hate you! None of us liberated women is supposed to admit that this condition exists at all, let alone that we understand it or – perish the thought – suffer from it.' Her perception of the feminist derision of masochism as a term of opprobrium at best and as a mechanism of female sub-jugation at worst is undoubtedly accurate. However, defined as a self-defeating personality type rather than as a sexual perversion or vehicle of male oppression, it has widespread application. To my understanding it cannot be dismissed as irrelevant to women's place in modern society. Neither can it be ignored as a source of considerable suffering.

Given the fact that all of us are inadequately mothered to some degree, all of us possess a greater or lesser capacity for maso-chistic behaviour as adults. We have only to look at the shelves of our local bookshops for confirmation of this observation. Contemporary female psychologists and novelists are almost obsessed by the urge to define mother–daughter–granddaughter relationships, their differing types and pathologies. As con-sumers in large numbers, we buy these books to help us under-stand our own personalities and problems. Most of these books deal with the problem of insufficient or incompetent maternal love, the anger of daughters and often the acting-out of that anger by granddaughters. Though they would blush to admit it, many authors deal with masochism.

Because masochism is in theory universal, we must all be honest enough and brave enough to examine its impact on our individual life histories and personalities, if we are to discover our own patterns of suffering. I, for one, have exhibited several of the hallmarks of masochism more times than I would care to admit over the years. I have occasionally lavished my attention and energy on activities which are neither immediately stimulating nor ultimately rewarding. I have routinely ignored opportunities for pleasure and later regretted it. I have sometimes been depressed. Although I am not trapped in an ever repeating pattern of self-defeating activities, I have nevertheless committed the same masochistic acts many times. Even worse, as the mother of a teenager, I increasingly appreciate the impact of my own deficiencies in mothering on my son.

These failures to love and be loved properly are matters of concern, but they are not causes of alarm or embarrassment. They are evidence not so much of gross pathology as of my inextricable bondage to the human condition and of my role in the repetition of imperfectibility generation by generation. They cause pain for me and my family. There is no apparent escape. There is, however, a spiritual medicine which relieves the pain and goes a long way towards curing the basic condition. It is divine love.

The heart of the Christian message – and the ultimate source of healing – is God's love for us. Having created us, he loves us as his children and as friends of his Son, Jesus Christ. Even more remarkably, he loves us for who we are, not for what we do. Our status as the beloved is secure in relationship to the Trinity. God is our father, Jesus is our friend and the Holy Spirit is our guide, encourager and comforter. Our great challenge is to accept as our own this eternal, heavensent identity as the beloved. We are invited to affirm that God loved us enough to create us, that Jesus loved us enough to die for us and that the Holy Spirit loves us enough to be our constant companion. How much more love do we mortals want and need, or should we desire?

It is in plumbing the depths of our relationship with God as Creator, Redeemer and Sanctifier that we compensate for the inadequacies of our particular human experiences of family relationships. Significantly, this trinitarian love enables us to love ourselves. It frees us to take full account of our strengths and weaknesses and to value ourselves properly. The striking difference between human love and divine love is its nature. God's love – unlike the love offered by parents, children, spouses and friends – is unconditional. We don't deserve it, and we most certainly haven't earned it. He loves us individually and uniquely, simply because of our relationship to him.

I, for one, find this stupendously generous love infinitely consoling in theory, but for years I found it difficult to accept in practice. When younger I was trapped by what one very close friend calls 'the achievement heresy', the notion that we have to earn love and respect by extraordinary performances in all of life's varied activities and that we are worth nothing if we fail to achieve first class honours in each and every endeavour. I knew that my parents basically loved me whatever I did, but I nonetheless felt powerfully compelled to win demonstrations of approval by presenting them with good school marks, flawless piano recitals and above average performances in other activities. My relationship with God was much the same. Although I believed that he loved me without regard to my performance of specific acts of piety, I sang in the choir, served in the junior altar guild, made bread for church bake sales and joined in appropriate charitable activities. I was the classic overachiever.

It is only in middle age and after a bout of herpes simplex encephalitis that I have begun to trust in God's love and to relax a bit. For months after contracting chickenpox and then encephalitis I was hardly able to lift my head, to concentrate clearly or do much of anything for anyone. Through this period of suspension from normal daily activities I was forced to learn a new mode of existing. I discovered a sense of time which resembled eternity far more than the earthly clock. I learned to listen to the sounds of birds and trees, to lose myself in the scent of flowers, to float in the sunshine and be filled with happiness.

Profoundly, I realised that God loved me in this incapacitated condition as much as in the active one. As a result, I could love myself as well. Indeed, I realised that I was probably more lovable in this relaxed state than in my usual state of nervous overextension. What a sobering revelation this was, but what a liberation as well! I ceased to be a modern follower of Pelagius (a fourth-century heretic who urged Christians to earn salvation through good works). After recovering from the disease, I gradually took on more and more – far more than most people would consider sane – but I am no longer trying to prove anything or earn anything. For the most part, I work for the challenge and pleasure. I have learned that I am quite good at some things and quite bad at many more. I can now smile at my successes and usually chuckle at my failures. As I become increasingly accepting of my limitations of talent and disposition, my self-love grows.

If the love of the Trinity enables us sooner or later to love ourselves, it also allows us, and indeed obliges us, to love others because they, too, are God's children. It is no accident that the first great commandment, 'to love the Lord thy God with all thy heart, with all thy soul and with all thy might', is quickly followed by the second, 'to love thy neighbour as thyself', for the litmus test of a loving relationship with God is a loving disposition towards other people. As God's children and Christ's friends we are bidden to display what Benita Kyle of the Westminster Pastoral Foundation calls Jesus' 'infinite regard for the other'. By this she means an immediate acceptance of the other person and a limitless concern for his wellbeing. This caring regard is quiet, dispassionate and deeply felt. It eschews both the desire to change the other person and the need to turn him or her into an object of charity.

In both my experience and observation Christians find the

injunction to love other people as ourselves particularly difficult. We frequently fall into the 'little Jack Horner' syndrome.
Intent on providing material and moral support to the needy
in body, mind and spirit, we give generously of whatever is
needed and then stand back in self-satisfaction and conclude
'my, what a good boy am I'! The sin is not just the shot to the
ego, but even more damagingly, the quickness to cast those
whom we help as recipients of our largesse rather than as individuals with their own need to give as well as receive. Like
masochists we keep a tight grip on the relationship, ensuring
that they remain ever grateful and that we remain the lords
and ladies bountiful.

As a graduate student I stepped into little Jack Horner's
corner on a weekly basis. Every Thursday night I set off to the
Home for Aged Women in Boston to see four impoverished
ladies over the age of eighty. Three were remarkable, feisty
characters who displayed a grim determination to remain fit
and avoid the infirmary, which no one seemed to leave except
in a coffin. The fourth, who had been a talented artist, was dis-
tressingly mentally disordered. None received many friends, so
my visits must have provided some amusement and companionship. I was humbled by their courage, but I spoiled the
entire venture by displaying a nauseating regard for my
worthiness in adding these visits to a busy academic schedule.

After two years of this deeply unattractive ego-stroking, my
complacency was shattered by visiting another 'shut in', a
woman who had been abandoned as a child, who had been
crippled by polio and who had recently overcome years of being
an alcoholic. She and I became friends – real friends. We were
both in leg irons and on crutches. She knew far more about
pain than I did, and she displayed a quiet dignity which the
healthy often missed but which others in pain instantly recognised and admired. She called me her little sister, and I was
deeply honoured. She taught me about being a human being,
about coming down from my pedestal and relating as an equal
to her friends, whose lives had been diminished from childhood

by disease, poverty and loneliness. It was a long fall from my pinnacle of privilege. It shattered my pride and turned me into someone who could relate to others with greater ease and with far more respect, someone who could receive love, not just give charity.

Divine love overcomes masochism not only by enabling us to love ourselves and our neighbours and to receive love in return, but also by enabling us to relinquish control over relationships. It frees us from the compulsion to protect ourselves as adults from being rejected and unsupported as we were to a greater or lesser degree as infants and toddlers. At one end of the scale are those like anorectics, who feel so threatened by others that they retreat into an isolated world in which they subdue themselves, sometimes to the point of death. At the other end are most of us, who are more frustrated than threatened by other people. We are tempted not so much to escape from family and friends into our own private world, where we reign supreme, as to wage a subtle but relentless battle for domination in close relationships to ensure that our needs are met, no matter what the consequences for those around us.

The key question in relationships, as in the rest of life, is who is in charge. The masochist in each of us votes for ourselves at all times and in all circumstances, for surrender could mean pain. I have long favoured one subtle but lethal weapon to keep others in their places. It is to impute guilt. If someone does not perform as I would wish, the best retaliation is to make him or her squirm upon being informed of the sin of omission. By imputing guilt I can subtly manipulate the other person into a disadvantaged position and seize control of the relationship, at least for a while. I ensure that I am not rejected, but what hurt I inflict on the unfortunate recipient!

Years ago one of the friends to whom this book is dedicated realised how much damage we were doing to our friendship by trying to control each other through guilt. She identified the 'tone of voice game' skilfully played by both of us to reduce the other to seething fury by making her feel guilty about not being as helpful or supportive as desired. The game consisted in communicating displeasure not so much through words as through a tone of deep disappointment. Her remedy was to suggest that when one of us did a good deed for the other, we refrain from saying, 'I hope she appreciates this' and instead say, 'I hope this gives her pleasure'. This simple substitution eliminated the playing fields on which we had previously waged the tone of voice game. It challenged us to become direct in stating our need for help and in expressing our gratitude. It is safe to predict that had we continued to behave like masochists bent on self-protection and control, our friendship would have disintegrated thirty years ago.

Slowly but surely I have realised the wisdom of treating others as God has treated me. This has meant abandoning the masochistic drive to control others. It has entailed praying for the grace to love others as I am loved by God, to support them as I am supported and to forgive them as I am forgiven. It has led me to begin to accept others as I wish to be accepted – warts and all. It has helped me see that what irritates me most in them is often what irritates me most in myself. It has encouraged me to list my own sins of omission and commission if I begin to claim the high moral ground and criticise their behaviour. It has guided me towards greater humility and increased compassion. I have a very long way to go, but at least I see the path of escape from the dead end road of masochism.

Chapter Ten

St Thérèse of Lisieux's 'Little Way'

WE NOW TURN to guidance offered by two well known and widely admired saints. St Thérèse of Lisieux instructs us in her 'little way' through pain, and St Teresa of Avila teaches us the great contemplative way. I rehearse their life stories in some detail, for every step of their journeys yields valuable insights into creative suffering and practical measures for us to follow.

The iconography of modern religious art – and even more especially cheap folk art – has consigned Thérèse of Lisieux to a world of sentimental piety where she most certainly does not belong. Plaster statues of the 'little flower of Lisieux', clutching a bunch of roses in one hand and smiling heavenward as she scatters rose petals with the other hand, repel Protestants who do not know her real story as well as Roman Catholics of an intellectual disposition. Agnostics and atheists, condemning her for displaying all that is superficial and deplorable in Christian spirituality, dismiss her without a second thought.

Beneath the sugary-sweet surface lay a woman of steel. Seven popes have revered her, one calling her 'a great man' and another 'the greatest saint of the twentieth century'.[1] A woman of unsuspected stature, she died of tuberculosis at the age of twenty-five. Hers was a prolonged, agonising death, endured with heroic fortitude after a decade of escalating emotional and physical suffering.

There was nothing overtly remarkable about Thérèse's life. Born into a petit bourgeois family in 1873, she entered the Carmelite convent at Lisieux in 1888. Endorsing the standards of rural society and the restraints of the Carmelite regime, she conformed to both unwaveringly. Her determination to fulfil all the expectations of family and religion – however petty or unreasonable – created an outwardly very ordinary life. Indeed, a few months before her death, one of her sisters at Carmel observed: 'Our Sister Thérèse of the Child Jesus will soon be dead, and I really can't imagine what Reverend Mother will find to say about her once she is gone. It won't be easy for her, I can tell you; for this little sister, charming as she is, has certainly never done anything worth the telling.'[2] It was not until after her death, when the various manuscripts she had written for her mothers superior were published, that her genius was revealed. Thérèse's rigid conformity to the dictates of family and religious order did not hamper that genius. On the contrary, it provided the foundation for it by forcing her to search her uneventful everyday home life, her convent cell, and finally the infirmary for a road to heaven. By outwardly pursuing the mundane and unexceptional, she reached emotional maturity and attained an extraordinary degree of spiritual awareness. She also discovered a meaning to her intense physical suffering.

To appreciate the landmarks along Thérèse's pathway through pain, it is necessary to penetrate the society in which she lived and to whose values she so slavishly ascribed. Rural French towns in the 1870s were light years away from cities in Britain and America at the turn of the twenty-first century. They were stable and tranquil. The Roman Catholic Church reigned supreme, providing an annual cycle of feasts and fasts by which everyone charted his life from the cradle to the grave and, even more fundamentally, supplying a moral and ethical code to which virtually all inhabitants subscribed. The Church also offered educational, medical and social services in addition to the obvious religious ones.

Into this world of piety and predictability Thérèse was born amidst comfort if not affluence. Her father was a watchmaker and jeweller who prospered in the little Norman town of

Alençon. Her mother was a lacemaker who employed local women to produce the intricately-worked table cloths and wedding veils which have made the town world famous. Before her parents married both sought to become religious, the father a Carthusian monk, the mother a Benedictine nun. Both were rejected. Undaunted, they turned their home into a kindergarten for the next generation of religious. Unfortunately but not unusually two sons (dedicated at birth as missionaries) died in infancy, as did two daughters; but the remaining five girls lived to become brides of Christ. Their childhood revolved around early morning mass, midday family prayers and evening devotional readings. Sunday was hallowed as a day of rest and meditation. For entertainment the father went fishing and bestowed his catch on the local Franciscan nuns while the mother wrote letters recording the activities of her children, thereby providing posterity with valuable information about Thérèse's earliest years.

Almost inevitably Thérèse's vocabulary of experience was entirely religious. Her first word is reported by her mother to have been 'heaven'.[3] This statement was perhaps more apocryphal than real, but it is nonetheless revealing of both the all-pervading religious atmosphere of the Martin household and of parental expectations. Thérèse's favourite childhood game was to build altars in the house and garden with tiny vases and candlesticks given as special presents by servants and family alike.

All of the five surviving Martin sisters were destined for the convent. But Thérèse was groomed for an extraordinary mission – to become a saint. As a little girl she was put on a pedestal at home, idolised by her father as his 'little queen' and pampered as the youngest child. Yet she was also projected by her older sisters to the highest mode of Christian existence.[4] Thérèse accepted their dream as her own. 'Reflecting then that I was born for glory, and searching for the means to attain it,' she later observed, 'it was inwardly revealed to me that my own glory would . . . consist in becoming a saint. This desire might seem full of temerity, but I still feel the same audacious confidence that I shall become a great saint'.[5] (The underlining is hers.)

Thérèse's singlemindedness in becoming a saint seems to us as breathtaking as her candour in proclaiming it. Her remarkable goal was, however, acceptable – if exceptional – in the devout provincial society of Lisieux. It was nurtured assiduously by the Martin family, yet it nonetheless posed a huge challenge for the girl. Thérèse was eager to please but not spineless, devout but not witless. Although she burst into tears of contrition and begged forgiveness whenever she erred and strayed from what was expected of her, she had a strong will of her own. Her mother noted in exasperation that she was 'so tiny, such a mad-cap, a very intelligent child, but much less docile than her sisters, and, above all, of an almost invincible obstinacy'.[6] Years later the Sub-Prioress at the convent testified that she was 'a little goody-goody to whom you would give communion without sending her to confession, but as artful as a wagon-load of monkeys. Mystical, comical: everything by turns.'[7] A far more complicated and attractive personality than the vapid smile on the plaster statue suggests, she endured horrific suffering in the pursuit of sanctity.

Thérèse charted three stages in her growth in holiness. Each instructed her in the school of pain. The initial period encompassed her earliest childhood, four years of peace and security when the family was all together and Thérèse was its little 'Benjamine et petite reine'.[8] This idyll came to an abrupt end in 1877 when Mme Martin died of breast cancer. Thérèse was old enough fully to appreciate her mother's unique role in the family and to experience a profound sense of grief.

The second phase of Thérèse's development in sanctity began a few months after Mme Martin's death. The devastated M. Martin moved his young family to Lisieux to be near his brother and sister-in-law and their two little girls (one of whom would follow the Martin sisters into the local Carmelite convent). In a large, comfortable house called Les Buissonnets,

The Shrubbery, overstuffed with heavy mahogany furniture and religious pictures, Thérèse spent her formative years. These were filled with sorrow and frustration.

The most harrowing event was the departure of her sister, Pauline, to the Carmelite convent when Thérèse was nine. As so often happened when mothers routinely died young, Pauline, the eldest daughter, had assumed adult responsibilities and had become Thérèse's second mother. Pauline was old enough to be maternal but young enough to be a close friend and confidante as well. The day she left Les Buissonnets for the convent, Thérèse's world fell apart. 'I was going to lose my mother all over again,' she wailed.[9] Shaking and trembling, Thérèse was sent to bed for months. There she hallucinated that nails on the walls were charred fingers. She slept fitfully, tormented by nightmares. Finally she became so disoriented that she failed to recognise her sisters.[10] Thérèse's doctors despaired of finding a remedy, but their failure was of no consequence. Her cure was delivered suddenly, unexpectedly and miraculously by the Virgin Mary in a vision. Recounting this remarkable experience, Thérèse admitted that

> there was no help, it seemed, for poor Thérèse on earth so I turned towards the [bedside statue of Mary], and all my heart went out into a prayer that my Mother in Heaven would have pity on me. All at once, she let me see her in her beauty, a beauty that surpassed all my experience – her face wore such a look of kindness and of pity as I can't describe. . . . With that, all my distress came to an end; two big tears started up from my eyes, and ran softly down my cheeks; but they were tears of joy, unadulterated joy.[11]

Thérèse's tears alerted her frantic sisters that she had regained her senses and that the crisis was over. However, despite restored health, the pain of separation from Pauline remained intense.

Thérèse realised that the only way to recover daily visits to Pauline and advance towards sanctity was to enter the convent as quickly as possible. The fact that she was only nine seemed irrelevant! Both Pauline and M. Martin supported her remarkable aspiration, but Marie de Gonzague, the Mother Superior, dismissed the proposal as preposterous and advised her to reapply when she turned sixteen. As ever when disappointed, Thérèse burst into uncontrollable sobs and determined to find a way around the obstacle.

Her first hope lay in the Bishop of Bayeux, whom she visited with her father to make a formal plea and for whom she arranged her hair in an adult chignon. Neither fooled nor persuaded, the Bishop endorsed the Superior's verdict, and Thérèse's eyes predictably brimmed with tears. Undeterred, she and her father set off with a band of pilgrims to Rome, where Thérèse seized the opportunity of a group audience with the Pope to breach protocol and implore the Holy Father to intercede for her. Before the Pope could respond, M. Révérony, the Bishop of Bayeux's long-suffering assistant, frantically rehearsed the arguments against her entry. Leo XIII

> fixed his eyes on me, and said, emphasising every syllable as he uttered it: 'All's well, all's well; if God wants you to enter, you will'. . . . His kindness gave me courage, and I wanted to go on; but the two members of the noble guard, finding that I paid no attention to their ceremonial touch, took me by the arms, and M Révérony helped them to lift me up; I kept my arms on the Pope's knee, and they had to carry me away by main force.[12]

M. Révérony was furious with Thérèse for being so outrageously defiant. But Thérèse rejoiced that he showed signs, from then on, 'of being at last convinced about my vocation'. (Only a fool could have been blind to her zeal.) She correctly reckoned that he had become a useful ally in swaying Marie de Gonzague to change her mind.[13]

Thérèse's second period of development came to an unexpected climax on Christmas Day, 1886. As with every milestone in her life, she imbued an ordinary event with extraordinary significance and spiritual meaning. Upon returning from midnight mass, she raced downstairs to open the presents which, according to the French custom, her father had arranged in her slippers. Reaching the door, she overheard him moan to an older sister that this was the last year he would perform such a childish ritual. Instantly she began to cry. But for the first time in her life she stopped herself, dried her eyes, put on a smile and ran into the room as if she had heard nothing. Laughing and hugging her father, she seized her slippers and treated him to a display of gratitude and love which assured him that his efforts had been worthwhile. For Thérèse this scene was nothing less than a 'complete conversion', the moment when her childhood ended. 'Our Lord had changed me', she proudly announced, 'into a different person.'[14] Surrendering the egocentricity of youth, she vowed thereafter to subordinate her every wish and action to others in the name of Jesus. This decision marked her first big step towards sanctity, and she knew it.

The third and last phase of her short life – encompassing her ten years in the convent – was a time of intense suffering. In 1888 Marie de Gonzague finally relented to pressure from the Martin family and M. Révérony and allowed Thérèse to enter the convent a year earlier than decreed. Leaving the comforts of Les Buissonnets with all its earthly delights, Thérèse embraced the austere life of the Carmelites.

In the bleak surroundings of the Lisieux convent she learned how – and even more importantly why – to suffer. Stomach aches and bronchial infections attacked her immediately; and in the spring of 1896 tuberculosis struck in all its horror. By then Thérèse was well educated in suffering. She had learned how to endure emotional torment before the physical agony began. This was crucial not only to the success of her own battle with pain, but also to the evolution of her guidance on living with suffering. We find these directions in *Story of a Soul*, her eminently sane and simply written autobiography. Subsequently edited a hundred times and translated into thirty-five languages, it has been read from England to China and is to this day the most popular religious book in France except for the Bible.

Like every convent-educated schoolgirl, Thérèse upheld the ideas of suffering offered in standard books of Christian piety. Among the most readily available were Thomas à Kempis's *Imitation of Christ* and St Francis de Sales's *Introduction to the Devout Life*, written in 1609 by the Bishop of Geneva.[15] Although the first was addressed specifically to monks and the second generally to lay men and women, both were often published, widely circulated and universally popular. What Thérèse made of them was, however, unique.

From Thomas à Kempis Thérèse derived the fundamental notion of suffering as the way of the cross and the highway to heaven. Thérèse bore not one cross, but two, in her ten years at the Lisieux Carmel. Had she not become masterful at carrying the first – rejection – she would not have been able to bear the second – excruciating physical pain – when it fell on her so suddenly and heavily.

Thérèse picked up the cross of rejection the moment she entered the convent in April 1888. It was handed to her by no less a person than the Mother Superior, Marie de Gonzague. An aristocratic authoritarian cursed with an aloof manner, Marie de Gonzague treated Thérèse harshly for an excellent reason. She explained it to the new postulant on her first day at Carmel:

> You are very young to be here, but you showed a determination beyond your years. However, you will find it much harder than you expect. I notice that your sisters still tend to treat you very much as a child – as the baby of the family. That is not how I shall treat you. If you are old enough to test your vocation here, and if we find that you have a vocation, then you are old enough to be treated like everyone else.[16]

Favouritism wreaks havoc in a religious community. Marie

de Gonzague rightly tried to prevent Pauline and Marie (soon to be joined by Céline Martin and cousin Marie Guerain) from lavishing special affection on their youngest relation. But she became obsessive in her campaign to topple Thérèse from the family pedestal. She subjected her to relentless and often undeserved attacks of criticism. For a girl whose greatest desire was to please, these assaults were devastating. With her usual wry sense of humour Thérèse observed: 'God saw to it that [Marie de Gonzague] should treat me very severely . . . I hardly ever met her without having to kiss the ground in penance for something I had done wrong.'[17] But Thérèse was fortified by Thomas à Kempis's dictum that 'the truly patient man takes no thought from what man, whether from his Superior, or from some equal or inferior . . . that his trial comes, but . . . he accepts the whole gratefully from the hand of God and counts it immense gain.'[18] Daily she subdued her will to God's through his most irascible vicegerent, Marie de Gonzague, and turned humiliation to her spiritual advantage.

While the challenge of bearing the Mother Superior's rejection overshadowed her entire life as a nun, rejection by other nuns, and apparent rejection by God as well, occurred early in her career. Rejection by the community came in 1890 when her father collapsed into madness. Today we accept mental illness as a distressing but common disease which affects many of us, but a century ago the people of rural France displayed far less tolerance. Pre-Freudian society suspected a lurking lunacy in all family members of an afflicted person and shunned them accordingly. Louis Martin, having recovered from two partially paralytic strokes, suffered a succession of emotional breakdowns between 1890 and his death in 1893. Confined to an asylum in Caen, he became increasingly deranged. For the Martin sisters his illness was a cause not only of distress but also of shame. In her autobiography Thérèse briefly mentioned their intense embarrassment and humiliation but quickly drew a curtain over the entire painful episode. 'I'm not going to try and describe what [my] feelings were: words couldn't do justice to them.'[19]

The period of M. Martin's 'cruel torment' and community aloofness was also a time of acute spiritual desolation for the young nun. Just when she most needed the solace of God's love, he seemed to disappear and leave her 'robbed of all consolation. . . . Dryness in prayer became a daily experience with me,' she confessed.[20] The convent became an emotional desert. Yet throughout her rejection she searched for – and found – a hidden grace. Because suffering enabled her to learn humility, 'the bitterest cup He puts to my lips always tastes delicious'.[21] Quoting Thomas à Kempis, she added: 'To suffer and remain unnoticed, that was all I longed for.'[22]

Thérèse translated Thomas à Kempis's fifteenth-century message into a very simple, modern idiom and called it 'the little way'. It stands in sharp contrast to the ways trodden by other famous saints whom she admired: martyrdom (to which she was attracted in all its lurid drama), priesthood (an interesting mode of sanctity for a Roman Catholic nun to contemplate a century ago) and scholastic achievement (inaccessible to a woman untutored in theology). 'Obviously, there's nothing great to be made of me,' she lamented, but with the crucial proviso:

> so it must be possible for me to aspire to sanctity in spite of my insignificance. I've got to take myself just as I am, with all my imperfections: but somehow I shall have to find out a little way, all of my own, which will be a direct short-cut to heaven. After all (I said to myself) we live in an age of inventions. Nowadays, people don't even bother to climb the stairs – rich people, anyhow; they find a lift more convenient. Can't I find a lift which will take me up to Jesus, since I'm not big enough to climb the steep stairway of perfection?[23]

Searching for biblical guidance, she found the answer in the

Book of Proverbs, which bids us all to be like children in relation to our heavenly father and to be ever loving and ever trusting. Here was Thomas à Kempis's thought couched in homey language. Like children we must accept whatever comes, either pain or pleasure, because we love and trust the Person who sends it. We find peace here and now if we conform our wills to his. We will also reach heaven after death when, in response to our lifetime of humble adoration, God will lift us in his arms and carry us straight to his kingdom, providing a divine lift! This simple formula for sanctity may sound literally puerile. But it is quite the opposite. It demands true heroism – albeit of a sort which all of us can display – as Thérèse herself soon discovered.

If Thomas à Kempis showed Thérèse how to deal positively with rejection, Francis de Sales taught her how to offer her suffering to God for the benefit of others. Whereas Thomas à Kempis focused on the small enclosed world of the monastery and the smaller world of the individual soul, de Sales the bishop gazed out at the secular world. He addressed his book to Philothea ('God-lover' in Greek), an imaginary Christian who was devout but not zealous.

Francis de Sales developed the broad theme that Christianity is a social religion in which every soul must work for the wellbeing of others. Unlike Thomas à Kempis, who conceived the soul's progress to heaven as an exclusively individual journey, de Sales regarded it as a corporate experience in which individuals find holiness through their membership of the Christian community and through the demands of ordinary life. Thomas à Kempis bade the monk to embark on an intense battle whose rigours might leave him useless to his fellow monks, while de Sales cautioned moderation in self-denial and restraint from any spiritual exercises which might deprive Christians of the physical energy and emotional reserves to live amicably and resourcefully with their neighbours. Wear a hair shirt occasionally or not at all, he advised, if it makes you unduly irritable with others. Eat whatever is put in front of you rather than fast, for deprivation of choice is a better penance than total refusal of nourishment, because it leaves you fit for service to others.[24] The animating force of all your thoughts and actions must be love, he commanded, for this is the cardinal virtue to which all others are subservient. Since 'charity alone can establish us in perfection', nuns like any other Christians must subordinate themselves to others in love and service.[25]

Having absorbed the wisdom of both Thomas à Kempis and Francis de Sales, Thérèse made the most important decision of her life. It was to offer her suffering in love for the benefit of others. Fulfilling this vocation, she would meet Christ's dual injunction to love God and her neighbour, not as an emotional reaction to God or individuals, but rather as an act of will. This commitment would entail a lifetime's vigilance to ascertain what was required in every waking moment, both in terms of her own sacrifice and in terms of the needs of others. It would require much thought, much prayer and even more grace, for she fully appreciated the huge discrepancy between what she wished to do and what she so often achieved. The task would be arduous but in the end successful, for she was convinced that with the lever of prayer saints 'shift the world'.[26] She resolved to become a saint by changing the world and those who live in it through the mighty force of sacrificial love.

To illustrate her new mission she hit upon the sentimental analogy of scattering prayers for lost souls like rose petals. Despite our embarrassment if not revulsion at this cloying image, we must put it into proper context. It derived from the tradition of children marching at the head of royal, church and wedding processions with baskets of flower petals in hand, strewing the way for monarchs, clerics and brides to follow. 'This love of mine, how to shew it?' she enquired.

> Love needs to be proved by action. Well, even a little child can scatter flowers, to scent the throne-room with their fragrance. . . . That shall be my life, to scatter flowers – to miss no single opportunity of making some small sacrifice

> . . . and doing it for love. I shall suffer all that I have to
> suffer – yes, and enjoy all my enjoyments too – in the
> spirit of love, so that I shall always be scattering flowers
> before your throne; nothing that comes my way but shall
> yield up its petal in your honour.[27]

Though expressed in off-putting imagery, Thérèse's theme was
identical to that of George Herbert, whose poetry has appealed
to the Anglo-Saxon disposition for three hundred years: 'I got
me flowers to straw thy way; I got me boughs off many a
tree.'[28]

For the first five years of her life as a nun her suffering
included a variety of minor tribulations as well as the serious
trials of rejection. Some, like a constant succession of stomach
aches and sore throats, came unbidden. They were nonetheless
welcomed as opportunities to offer vexations to the Almighty
for his infinitely higher purposes. Others were courted, and
these are perhaps more instructive of Thérèse's determined
pursuit of the holy in the ordinary. One of the best illustrates
an easily missed opportunity to subdue one's will for the benefit of another. It also provides an excellent example of
Thérèse's shrewdness in assessing the human condition. How
should you respond, she asked, to those who irritatingly display 'want of judgement, want of education, the touchiness you
find in certain people's characters, which spoil the amenities of
life', i.e. your own enjoyment of it? Since 'moral disabilities of
this kind are chronic,' she lamented, 'there's no real hope of
curing them.'[29] The answer lies in singling out those who are
least attractive, 'roadside casualties who need a good
Samaritan. Often just a word or a friendly smile are enough to
make these difficult natures open out.'[30]

At other times a sympathetic gesture is necessary but
almost impossible to extend. As an example, Thérèse
rehearsed the tale of an arthritic older sister who needed help
getting from the chapel to the refectory every evening for
supper. 'A trifling service,' she commented,[31] but one which
cost a fortune in patience. The elderly nun was clumsy,

impatient and ungrateful, a woman who hated to be dependent and expressed her frustration by endlessly carping at
those who tried to help her. Everyone at Lisieux smartly
backed away from this prickly sister. Thérèse, therefore,
decided that the modest terrain from the chapel to the refectory
would be an admirable frontier for offering her own sacrifice of
rejection, anger and perhaps even love, should she ever find
the grace to be truly affectionate towards this tiresome old
woman.

Her resolution launched a daily battle. It began in frustration and defeat, for Thérèse could not easily quell her dislike of
the nun and the task she had set herself. But after several
months it ended in the triumph of Thérèse over herself.
Gradually, she acquired the ability to absorb acid comments
without resentment or anger. All the while she kept smiling,
providing whatever was needed and eventually maintaining a
posture of genuine compassion.

A second homey example arose when another nun drove
Thérèse to distraction during hours of silent meditation with
the irritating habit of clicking her tongue as she ruminated in
prayer. At first Thérèse tried to ignore her, but this was

> absolutely useless; there was I with the sweat pouring
> down me, in the attempt to make my prayer into a prayer
> of mere suffering! Suffering – but somehow I must get rid
> of the nervous irritation, and suffer peaceably, joyously;
> that is, with peace and joy deep down in my soul. So I hit
> on the idea of trying to like this exasperating noise,
> instead of trying vainly not to hear it. I devoted myself to
> listening hard, as if the sound were that of some delight-
> ful music, and all my prayer – it certainly wasn't the
> prayer of quiet! – consisted in offering this music to our
> Lord.[32]

In other myriad unobserved episodes like these Thérèse
learned how to transform the trials of daily living into a sacrifice to God. '[I]t was this way of suffering I had to follow,' she

pointed out, 'and yet there was no outward sign of it – perhaps it would have relieved my feelings a bit if other people had been conscious of it, but they weren't.'[33]

Thérèse decided that the beneficiaries of her sacrifices – both great and small – would be those in purgatory and those who had not yet embraced Christianity on earth. Her first 'catch' was a notorious murderer called Pranzini, who slit the throats of his wife, daughter and maid yet refused to admit guilt or display remorse. Like everyone else in France, Thérèse followed the trial with morbid fascination. But her titillation soon gave way to alarm when she realised that he would die in mortal sin and go to hell. Here was an ideal opportunity to test her new vocation as an intercessor. She prayed fervently that Pranzini would repent before it was too late. To her immense satisfaction she read in the paper several days after his execution that Pranzini had suddenly seized and kissed a crucifix moments before the guillotine had fallen, thereby opening to him the gates of heaven and to her a lifelong mission to save souls through prayer.[34]

Having experienced the thrill of 'sponsoring' a conversion, Thérèse set her heart on becoming a foreign missionary. It is most unusual for Carmelites to abandon their enclosures for the missionary field. But at the end of the nineteenth century French priests, intent on converting the inhabitants of French Indo-China, invited a small band of Carmelites to join them with a view to establishing a convent for devout Indo-Chinese women in Hanoi. Unexpectedly, Marie de Gonzague blessed Thérèse's application to go with them. At the last minute, however, Thérèse was forced to remain behind. Suddenly and irrevocably, she succumbed to tuberculosis. Here was the final unexpected and unwanted opportunity to accept God's will as her own. Without a murmur of dismay she realised that she must surrender her ambition to be a missionary and accept without complaint the less glamorous vocation of intercessor.[35]

In the role of intercessor she was stunningly successful. Indeed, she became a far greater luminary as an intercessor than she could ever have become as a missionary. Ordinands heading for the Orient in the 1890s enjoyed her prayerful support, and countless missionaries have prayed to her since her death and have felt the benefit of her patronage.[36] Their testimonies, many of which advanced her official beatification and sanctification, have made her the patron saint of foreign missionaries. To her evident satisfaction and delight Thérèse quickly recognised her clout both on earth and in eternity. She ascribed it to the potent combination of prayer, pain and sacrifice. 'Our Lord let me see clearly that if I wanted to win souls, I'd got to do it by bearing a cross; so the more suffering came my way, the more strongly did suffering attract me.'[37] This was not masochism. This was courage. It was the crucial link in Thérèse's spirituality which gave meaning to her pain, both emotional and physical. Defying the destructive nature of suffering, she learned to welcome pain as a lever to raise the banner of hope, redemption and generosity over her sickbed.

Fittingly, Thérèse's herculean struggle with physical pain began on Good Friday 1896. After the Maundy Thursday celebrations the night before, 'I went up to bed ... and I had scarcely laid my head on the pillow when I became conscious of what seemed like a warm tide that rose up, up, till it reached my lips. . . . [S]urely I must be spitting blood?'[38] The next morning she observed the rule of silence and told only the Mother Superior, whom she was obliged under the Carmelite rule to inform of any illness. She begged Marie de Gonzague to treat her as usual. The Superior readily assented. Not only did she allow Thérèse to continue to work and pray on schedule, she also deprived her of proper care as her condition steadily and visibly deteriorated over the next winter.[39]

A half century before the discovery of antibiotics there was no cure for tuberculosis. There were, however, known means of alleviating discomfort. These Marie de Gonzague denied the young nun in her zeal to avoid needless expense and to prevent the Martin sisters from making a fuss. She refused Thérèse a proper bland but nourishing diet, a warming fire in winter and even a soft comfortable bed.[40] A year after Thérèse first haemorrhaged, she could struggle no longer and finally retired to the infirmary. Coughing up blood daily depleted her strength, while increasing congestion and constriction in the lungs made breathing ever more difficult. As if this were not enough, she developed gangrene of the intestines, a common side effect of TB. This caused constant nausea, vomiting and dehydration as well as terrible pain. By July 1897 she could eat nothing, including communion wafers, and could inhale only shallow gasps of air. Cursed, as it were, with a strong constitution, she lingered in this excruciating state until 30 September. A week before she died a friend observed, 'Oh, what a terrible illness! How you must have suffered!' And Thérèse responded, 'Yes! What a mercy it is to have faith! If I didn't have faith, I should have killed myself without a moment's hesitation.'[41] These were dying words of the utmost realism and courage, not the platitudes normally associated with Thérèse, the plaster saint.

Faith kept her firm in her determination to suffer in love for the salvation of lost souls. But it provided no consolation. Like every other human being – including Jesus – she walked through the Valley of the Shadow of Death. Often she warned her watching sisters:

> Don't be upset, dearest sisters, if I suffer a great deal and if you see no sign of happiness in me when I reach the point of death. Our Lord too died a victim of love, and see what his death agony was like!
>
> Our Lord died on the cross in agony, yet his was the finest of deaths for love . . . The only example, indeed. Dying of love doesn't mean dying in transports of joy.[42]

Quite the opposite in fact. Like her Saviour, Thérèse felt utterly abandoned by God. She could no longer feel his presence, nor even believe that heaven awaited her. Knowing that she might be blaspheming, she nonetheless admitted that her faith in the hereafter had vanished. Ever since childhood, she ruefully observed,

> I had this feeling that a better country was to be, one day, my abiding home. And now, all of a sudden, the mists around me have become denser than ever; they sink deep into my soul and wrap it round so that I can't recover the dear image of my native country any more – everything has disappeared. I get tired of the darkness all around me, and try to refresh my jaded spirits with the thoughts of that bright country where my hopes lie; and what happens? It is worse torment than ever: the darkness itself [seems to say] 'It's all a dream, this talk of a heavenly country, bathed in light, scented with delicious perfumes, and of a God who made it all, who is to be your possession in eternity! You really believe, do you, that the mist which hangs about you will clear away later on? All right, all right, go on longing for death! But death will make non-sense of your hopes: it will only mean a night darker than ever, the night of mere non-existence.'[43]

With Christ on the cross she could cry, 'My God, my God, why have you forsaken me?'

When life's basic amenities – breath, strength and hope – had passed away, only one thing was left to Thérèse. That was her will. Deprived of comforts both earthly and heavenly, she nonetheless retained the faculty of choice. She determined to offer herself in dying, as in living, as a sacrifice of love to Love. It was the only choice which made sense in a world which had lost all meaning. Throughout her life she had worked hard to develop the habit of conforming her will to that of God, and the habit had mercifully become ingrained. Towards the end all she could repeat was that 'the only thing I want badly now is to go on loving til I die of love'.[44] From some mouths this would have been cant. On Thérèse's lips it was the distillation of a short lifetime's rugged campaign.

Steps towards canonisation were taken almost immediately

after her death on 30 September 1897. She was declared a saint in 1925. To advance her cause the Martin sisters overlaid her autobiography with statements of devotion which conformed to their particularly sucrose brand of piety and which they believed would attract a wider audience than Thérèse's terser prose. Local artisans began producing plaster casts of the 'little flower of Lisieux'. The town became a place of pilgrimage, and local purses bulged as her fame spread. Much of what was produced was tasteless and tawdry. Yet behind the commercialism and sentimentality lay a simple woman with a simple message. Both appealed not only to semiliterate French farmers but also to highly sophisticated men of academic distinction like Karl Rahner and Hans Urs von Balthasar, to spiritual giants like Thomas Merton and to practical holy women like Dorothy Day, the American social worker. Millions have accepted Thérèse's invitation to follow the 'little way' by offering their suffering on the altar of love for the benefit of others. In doing so they have found a pattern and purpose for their own pain as well as a means of attaining life eternal.

Before leaving the 'little way', it is imperative to point out its distortion and misapplication. Both have caused tremendous needless suffering. They have resulted from a misunderstanding of the nature of Christian sacrifice. Thérèse's prayerful suffering was a free will offering. She regarded it as the natural response of love and self-giving to a loving and self-giving God. She thus conceived her 'little way' as a means of imitating the Godhead. Practised on this heroic level, it was the noblest and most creative way possible to deal with pain.

One distortion of the 'little way' has occasionally been pursued in monasteries and convents. It has been adopted by superiors like Marie de Gonzague, who have imposed sacrifice on their communities. All superiors are required to enforce the rules of their particular community. Benedictines supervise a fairly gentle rhythm of work, rest and prayer, while Carthusians and Carmelites dictate a far more rigid and less comfortable regime. All monastic rules are tough to a degree.

But beyond that point there is an area of discretion open to the superior in deciding how to interpret the rule and how much stringency to impose. This is the area where cruelty can gain sway. It is possible for superiors to deprive communities of adequate creature comforts and sufficient emotional support. In doing so they make the lives of monks and nuns needlessly miserable. They impose suffering. They demand that brothers and sisters 'offer up' pain, frustration and natural rebellion against a destructive regime to God without complaint. They fail to recognise that coercion and cruelty are totally inimical to the true concept of Christian sacrifice. They lose sight of the voluntary nature of Christ's offering and of Thérèse's. They confuse sacrifice with oppression.

Another distortion has been developed among the laity since the publication of Thérèse's autobiography. In its most pronounced form it has been imposed on young girls by an unholy alliance of pious mothers and zealous priests. It has been derived from the cult of Thérèse as the model young female, who subdued her will totally to God by renouncing her own talents and tastes and by pursuing meekness, gentleness and patience as expressions of that submission. It has substituted passivity for vitality and a rigid conformity for individuality.

Like the monastic distortion of the 'little way' this distortion has been enforced by those in authority on the obedient. One example will illustrate their plight. Maria Filippetto, 'Maria of Padua' as she has become known, was an extremely bright and lively little girl who joined 'St Thérèse's Little Legion'. In the words of her hagiographer, 'from the age of three this marvellous child began a tremendous combat with her rebellious nature, which went on for years, until finally she became a sweet, smiling, gracious child, facing the most terrible suffering with an heroic courage such as recalls the virgin martyrs of the first ages'.[45] The top of her class at school, a pretty girl attracted to frilly frocks and a popular leader among her friends, she contracted diabetes during World War One, just before the discovery of insulin and with it a means of controlling this fatal disease. Both her mother and parish priest insisted that she imitate Thérèse as a 'victim to Divine Love'. She readily assented. Withstanding several operations without anaesthesia and without complaint, she prayed constantly, succumbed slowly and all the while uttered pious statements like 'press, press still more our little cluster of grapes'.[46] When she died in 1925, her story was translated into every European language and was circulated in India, China, Japan, and the Americas as an inspiration to other devout little girls.

Maria of Padua, and those who emulated her, are undoubtedly paragons of virtue. But their sacrifice is a travesty of that offered by Thérèse. It conforms to a pattern of living and dying dictated by ecclesiastical and family figures. The loss of freedom rather than the magnitude of suffering born courageously is the issue. It is true that Thérèse's sisters implanted the idea of sanctity in their youngest sibling and after her death supported her beatification and canonisation. But it is equally clear and significant that Thérèse accepted their challenge and devised a unique 'little way' to meet it. No one imposed it on her. No one even knew she was pursuing it. Only after her death, when the full oeuvre of her writings was discovered and published, did her real holiness come to light. It is a light which others in pain can follow – voluntarily and unobtrusively – with incalculable benefit to themselves and others.

Chapter Eleven

Steps Through the Passing Moment

THE KEY TO creative suffering is to find God in the passing moment. Thérèse's 'little way', as we have seen, sanctifies the most mundane of events and experiences by transforming the stuff of ordinary living into a sacrament, 'an outward and visible sign of an inward and spiritual grace'. It enabled her to turn the convent and infirmary into a forecourt of heaven. Her 'little way' and the wider tradition of searching for God in the present moment from which it springs have much to offer those of us in chronic pain. They provide the surest way I know to change potentially life and soul-destroying suffering into a positive life-affirming and spiritually creative enterprise. They do not, I hasten to add, offer a sugar coating to the pill of suffering which protects the person in pain from experiencing in full the discomforts and distresses of his or her condition. They do, however, secure an effective means of swallowing the bitter pill with courage, hope and dignity.

Like millions of other Christians – including Thérèse – I learned about the sacrament of the here and now from Brother Lawrence, a seventeenth-century French monk. In 1693 his letters and conversations were collected into a little book entitled *The Practice of the Presence of God*, and like Thérèse's *Life of A Soul*, it became a perennial bestseller not only in France but throughout the Christian world.

Brother Lawrence was a simple peasant who as a youth was wounded in the leg while fighting in the French army against the Swedes.[1] Left with a permanent disability and unfit for military service, he became a footman to Monsieur de Fulbert, treasurer of the royal exchequer. His unsuitability for even this modest position became evident on a trip to Burgundy to purchase wine for the treasurer's cellar. With typical humour he described the episode to the Abbé Joseph de Beaufort, his faithful biographer, editor and publisher. The Abbé recounts that the shopping trip was 'a painful task for him as he had no aptitude for business, was lame in one leg, and could only get about the boat by rolling himself over the casks'![2] Fearing that he would upset the boat and lose the precious cargo of wine, Brother Lawrence 'told God that it was *his* business', resigned his post shortly thereafter and joined a Carmelite community in Paris in 1666.[3] Here he found great contentment over many years and discovered a totally unexpected vocation as a spiritual counsellor.

Brother Lawrence's correspondence with those who turned to him for advice was as wise as it was wide. His theme to one and all was simple and direct: 'Do everything for the love of God.'[4] As he observed to Abbé Joseph, 'it requires neither skill nor knowledge to go to God, but only a heart resolute to turn to him'.[5] Encouraging a sixty-four year old lady to 'make a start' and take 'courage', he pointed out that

> God does not ask much of us – an occasional remembrance, a small act of worship, now to beg his grace, at times to offer him our distresses, at another time to render thanks for the favours he has given. . . . It is not needful always to be in church to be with God. We can make a chapel of our heart, to which we can from time to time withdraw to have gentle, humble, loving communion with him. Everyone is able to have these familiar conversations with God, some more, some less – he knows our capabilities. . . . Perhaps he only waits for us to make one whole-hearted resolve![6]

To a sick mother superior he humbly advised: 'Offer him ceaselessly your sufferings. Beg him for strength to bear them. . . . Worship him in your infirmities. . . . I will aid you therein by my poor and puny prayers.'[7] Months before his own death in 1691 he again instructed her to 'be courageous. Make a virtue of necessity. Ask God, not to be delivered from the pains of the body, but for the strength to suffer with courage, for his love, all that he shall will, and for as long as it shall please him. . . . Love', he reminded her, 'sweetens sufferings.'[8]

Hours before Brother Lawrence's death a member of his community asked rather stupidly if he were in pain, and he responded emphatically: 'Pardon, *I am* in pain. The place in my side hurts. But my soul is content.'[9] Indeed, the pain was severe but it was not destroying him. Having sought God in all he had undertaken and endured for over twenty-five years as a monk, and having lovingly handed it all back to God day by day, he was able to face with equanimity life's greatest challenge: to offer himself to God at death as the supreme token of love in faith and hope.

My favourite English advocate of the sacrament of the present moment is the sublime seventeenth-century poet-cum-parson, George Herbert. His poem 'The Elixir' celebrates this sacrament.[10] Well known as a hymn as well as a poem, it relies on the most ordinary of household images alongside the less familiar ones of alchemy, an early modern pseudoscience based on magic. Its message is that by searching for God in all our tasks, we can find not only the grace to perform the job; we can also find God, and see his glory revealed in the most seemingly insignificant of activities.

> Teach me, my God and King,
> In all things thee to see,
> And what I do in any thing,
> To do it as for thee:
>
> Not rudely, as a beast,
> To runne into an action;
> But still to make thee prepossest,
> And give it his perfection.

In other words, do not rush into an action like a dumb animal but rather think of God first, perform the action as well as you humanly can and trust that God will perfect it.

> A man that looks on glasse,
> On it may stay his eye;
> Or if he pleaseth, through it passe,
> And then the heav'n espie.

Glass may be held in two ways. You can either use it like a mirror and see your own image, or you can look through it to see the sky and clouds. Even more importantly you, yourself, can 'passe' through the glass to heaven in that twinkling of an eye if only you keep God in mind.[11]

> All may of thee partake:
> Nothing can be so mean,
> Which with this tincture (for thy sake)
> Will not grow bright and clean.

The imagery here is that of alchemy insofar as the tincture is a cleaning agent, but the analogy is to the eucharist. Everyone can take holy communion; nothing is so humble; all can be cleansed, forgiven and redeemed through it.

> A servant with this clause
> Makes drudgerie divine:
> Who sweeps a room, as for thy laws,
> Makes that and th'action fine.

> This is the famous stone
> That turneth all to gold:
> For that which God doth touch and own
> Cannot for lesse be told.

Just as remembering God while working transforms the

common feat of cleaning a room into a sacred act, so God turns
the common elements of bread and wine into Christ's presence
in the eucharist. The 'famous stone' is the philosopher's stone
which was reputed by alchemists to turn base metal into pure
gold. Grace is like that stone. It is the means whereby God
'touch[es]' and 'own[s]' all creation and, in so doing, makes it
holy.[12] This is a meditative poem which merits slow reading,
pondering and memorising not only for pleasure but also for
frequent repetition and subtle programming of our deepest
desires.

I have discovered my own modest but effective way of celebrating the passing moment, thereby turning pain into grist
for the heavenly mill. Mine is a particular form of intercessory
prayer which resembles what Thérèse would have called 'reparation'. By that she would have meant not simply offering
her sufferings for the benefit of others but even substituting
her suffering on earth for the pains of hell which the un-
baptised in France and Indo-China would endure eternally,
just as Catherine of Siena had aimed at substituting her
earthly suffering for the purgatorial trials of her relations. 'I
have not chosen an austere life to expiate my own faults,'
Thérèse explained, 'but those of others.'[13]

Thérèse's aspiration was lofty, but I find it unattractive both
for what it seems to imply about God and for what it does to
human beings. It appears to rest on an image of an unmerciful
Deity who must be placated with sacrifices before he will dis-
pense grace, justice and healing. To my way of thinking, Jesus
atoned for the sins of humankind once and for all time. He was
the Lamb of God, to use biblical imagery, and his sacrifice is
sufficient for all people throughout the ages. We can add
nothing to this complete action save the metaphorical sacrifice
of praise and thanksgiving.

Besides suggesting incompleteness, Thérèse's notion of
reparation also holds pitfalls for those who pray. It views them
as superior to those for whom they pray by virtue of being
Christians, thus constructing an easy slide into the mire of

pride. And it casts them as sacrificial victims, hurling them potentially into the even murkier bog of masochism.

My concept of 'reparative' intercession avoids these obstacles. It bids me stand beside – not instead of – those for whom I pray. It is based on the realisation that all of us who suffer are united by an invisible bond of common experience and, hopefully, empathy. As in a Greek chorus, some of us voice the concerns of the entire body, often focusing our entreaties on one person representing the tragedy of the human condition. By praying this way we identify our corporate needs as expressed in individual suffering. We intercede in the hope that God will respond in love, bestowing healing of body or mind when he deems appropriate and supplying grace to endure and grow through suffering when he wishes to teach us that wholeness and health are not necessarily identical.

In my form of reparative intercession a stab of pain is the immediate reminder to pray. I hit upon this use of pain when a friend's son became very ill. She asked the six of us who had shared in an ecumenical prayer group every Monday evening for nine years to help her face the trauma of mental illness and to join her in supporting her son through whatever trials lay ahead.

As a first step the other members of the group decided to fast and pray for him on a particular day. Fasting was impracticable for me, as I was going through a bad patch in which I needed to take strong pain killers and to buffer them regularly with food. It occurred to me that I could join in the group's prayer by using the pain to remind me to pray for my friend's son. Every time I felt a jab or ache, I sent up a brief intercession on his behalf. My pain was instantly transformed into something positive and I was rewarded with three blessings. First, I was enabled to support my friend and her son in their distress. Second, I was relieved of my own sense of isolation in moments of pain. Third, I was led to recognise pain as an invitation to ask for grace, look through Herbert's glass 'and then the heav'n espie' and thus sanctify the passing moment.

For the past year I have been praying in this way for another friend's son who is displaying emotional problems. Sadly, I have relegated the first young man (who has stabilised) to my longer intercessory list. In my experience it is impossible to employ this special form of intercession for more than one person at a time, because this prayer must be an immediate, automatic response to the thrust of pain. It must be made without thought and without lingering. It must transpire in the passing moment, uniting you in seconds to the other person and through him or her to the pain of the cosmos. On good days you may offer this form of prayer only occasionally, while on bad days you may repeat it often. Although it can be practised by anyone in pain, it is best utilised by those in chronic pain, for its value seems to come from spontaneous repetition over long periods of time. The healthy are entirely disqualified from celebrating this particular sacrament of the passing moment!

From experience I know the sense of support imparted by intercessory prayer. There have been critical moments in my life – the difficult birth of my son, for example, and the fraught months following encephalitis – in which I have felt literally upheld by friends in prayer. Even more importantly, I have also been blessed with a happy outcome in times of acute distress through, if not entirely because of, the prayers of friends. On those occasions the alliance of divine and human will seems to create what might be called a 'butterfly effect'. The power of prayer compared to the heavy armaments of modern medicine may appear as infinitesimal as a butterfly's wing. Nevertheless, prayer seems to tip the balance of probabilities towards recovery by maximising the potential benefits of medicine and of caring support. Given its potency in promoting health, intercession may possibly be the greatest exercise of love which one human can undertake for another.

Both as the giver and as the beneficiary of intercessory prayer, I have come to regard the role of intercessor as an important 'vocation'. It is especially suited to the frail, the elderly, the chronically ill and all who are physically impeded from participating in life's full range of activities. By praying for their friends, families, parishes, the poor, the starving, the persecuted and the war-ravaged, intercessors may find a purpose and dignity to life which has been stripped of obligations and otherwise consigned to passivity.

I can think of one lady in particular who resides in the retirement home attached to All Saints Convent in Oxford. Despite her crippling and ever-worsening disabilities, she pursues a generous ministry of prayer for those whom she knows, for causes which she supports and for all who are commended to her by those of us who recognise her as a power-house of prayer. She is a model for us all. If in the years ahead I were to become permanently incapacitated, I would pray for the grace to emulate her compassion and find a steady voice in the mighty chorus of intercessors articulating the needs of suffering humanity.

Chapter Twelve

St Teresa of Avila's Great Way

TERESA OF AVILA is one of the most attractive people ever to be formally declared a saint. Energetic, imaginative, determined, full of common sense and good humour, she led both a very active and a very contemplative life. Between 1561 and 1582 she founded a reformed branch of the Carmelite order of friars and nuns and wrote the most popular books on contemplative prayer ever published. These were considerable achievements, ones which led her to embrace absolute poverty and to battle successfully with the Papacy, the Spanish monarchy and the Inquisition. All of these dramatic and well-recorded experiences came to her after fifteen years of crippling illness.

Much of Teresa's attraction for us lies in her very modern capacity to succeed in a country divided politically, socially and religiously. Early sixteenth-century Spanish society was as tumultuous as Europe today. The Moors had been expelled and Spain united under Ferdinand of Aragon and Isabella of Castile in 1492, but there was still a large population of Jewish converts to Christianity whose allegiance to the Roman Catholic Church was suspect. Teresa belonged to this group. In 1485 her grandfather confessed to practising Judaism in secret and repented in public before reaffirming his orthodoxy. Despite her father's conformity to the Church and his legal acquisition of noble status, Teresa inherited the taint of the *converso* (the 'converted').[1]

If Church authorities distrusted her Jewish lineage, they feared her espousal of private prayer even more. Direct

communication between God and the individual without benefit of sacraments dispensed by the Church was the hallmark of
the Protestant Reformation, which was launched by Martin
Luther when Teresa was four years old and was galvanised
into a political force which tore Europe apart when she was
thirteen.

Teresa's third and most obvious disability was simply being
a woman. The crowns of England, Scotland and the
Netherlands were worn by highly competent women in the sixteenth century, but the Church is a far more conservative insti-
tution than the State and to this day far less accepting of
women. Because she was a woman, Teresa was automatically
relegated to an inferior level in the ecclesiastical hierarchy.
She was also denied the education which would have qualified
her to write on prayer and reform her religious order without
excessive attention from the Inquisition. None of these dis-
advantages stopped her from attaining her goals, but all
generated obstacles which required ingenuity and stamina to
overcome.

Until the age of twenty-three Teresa was a healthy, high-
spirited and modestly pious young woman.[2] As a child she and
her brother played 'capture the Moors' in the garden. When
Teresa was seven, they stole provisions and set off down the
road from Avila towards Africa to slay real Moors for Christ. A
worried uncle apprehended them, realising that their zeal was
inspired partly by a laudable desire to win the martyr's crown
and partly by a flair for the dramatic fuelled by the romantic
novels which entertained their chronically-ill mother.

Several years later, after her mother's death, the teenage
Teresa alarmed her father by her coquettish behaviour and
provoked him to send her to a nearby convent to limit her
social life and advance her education. Teresa was not pleased.
Indeed, she was furious. The convent remained uncongenial to
her until she realised that the religious life rather than the
martyr's death would obtain the heavenly reward. After a prolonged battle against her love of worldly comforts and

pleasures she quelled her aversion to a nun's deprivations and entered the Carmelite Convent of the Incarnation at Avila in 1536. Heaven seemed assured. But her health began to deteriorate rapidly and dramatically.

It is extremely difficult – not to say risky – to diagnose the illness of a person who lived four hundred years ago. The understanding of physical and emotional states in the sixteenth century was primitive and the vocabulary of medicine extremely limited. Nevertheless, physicians of the twentieth century have felt fairly confident in diagnosing Teresa's malady. This is because she provides sufficiently detailed descriptions of her condition in her autobiography to support a well-informed guess. This evidence suggests that she suffered from catalepsy.

Catalepsy is a condition which results in partial paralysis. For eight months in 1539 Teresa was almost totally incapacitated. This illness began with what was apparently an epileptic seizure. In Teresa's own vivid words this

> fit lasted for four days, [when] I was in such a state that only the Lord can know what intolerable sufferings I experienced. My tongue was bitten to pieces; nothing had passed my lips; and because of this and of my great weakness my throat was choking me so that I could not even take water. All my bones seemed to be out of joint and there was a terrible confusion in my head.[3]

Catalepsy immediately followed the seizure or, possibly, series of seizures:

> As a result of the torments I had suffered during these days, I was all doubled up, like a ball, and no more able to move arm, foot, hand or head than if I had been dead, unless others moved them for me. I could move, I think, only one finger of my right hand. It was impossible to let anyone come to see me, for I was in such a state of distress that I could not endure it. They used to move me in a sheet, one taking one end and one the other.[4]

Once the acute state passed, she was able to get about on hands and knees like a crab. She maintained this awkward posture for nearly three years.

Unfortunately for Teresa, the various doctors employed by the convent and her family failed to relieve her anguish. In fact, their remedies did her far more harm than good, and on several occasions they nearly killed her. The standard arsenal of sixteenth-century medicine included bleeding, emetics and arsenic, all designed to lower the body's heat and balance its humours. Once again, Teresa's own words tell the story best. In one clinic she remained

> for three months, suffering the greatest trials, for the treatment was more drastic than my constitution could stand. At the end of two months, the severity of the reme-dies had almost ended my life. My strength suffered a grave decline, for I could take nothing but liquid and became so wasted, that after they had given me pur-gatives daily for almost a month, I was, as it were, so shrivelled up that my nerves began to shrink. These symptoms were accompanied by intolerable pain which gave me no rest by night or by day. Altogether I was in a state of great misery.[5]

More than once she became unconscious and was given up for dead. The sacrament of extreme unction was administered and her eyelids were sealed with wax in preparation for burial.

Today we realise that catalepsy can have psychological as well as organic origins. We can conjecture that Teresa's paraly-sis was primarily psychological. Had it been entirely organic, she would most probably not have recovered. The fact that Teresa did recover, albeit very slowly and painfully, indicates that the disease was generated and ultimately dispelled by emotions. In other words, it was what we would call today 'psychosomatic'. The muscular stiffness, spasms and atrophy as well as the paralysis were entirely real and legitimately alarming to her and those around her. To discover why she experienced them and why they spontaneously disappeared, we must look to her experiences between 1538, when she contracted the disease at the age of twenty-three, 1544 when she began to improve, and 1554 when she finally recovered at the age of thirty-nine. It was a prolonged agony.

Teresa's entrance to the Convent of the Incarnation at Avila in 1536 eighteen months before the onslaught of illness was fraught with guilt. Her mother had died nine years earlier, and Teresa had quite naturally centred her affections entirely on her father. In the custom of sixteenth-century Spanish children, she also respected him as head of the family and the author of all decisions regarding its members' welfare. Don Alonso fully reciprocated her love and expected her to remain at home as his companion.

When she begged her father to allow her to test her vocation as a nun, he adamantly refused and forbade her to seek entry to any convent before his death. This was an intolerable restraint on Teresa, who, distrusting her resolve and fearing that she would weaken if she waited that long, determined to embrace the religious life by stealth. Early in the morning of 2 November 1536, she sneaked out of her father's house and walked through the door of Avila's enclosed Carmelite convent. Don Alonso was distraught by her sudden and irrevocable departure. Teresa was equally shattered. 'When I left my father's house my distress was so great that I do not think it will be greater when I die,' she later lamented.[6]

Teresa's guilt at disobeying and deserting her father was compounded by the guilt which had earlier that year provoked her to enter the religious life. Like most late medieval and early modern Christians, she experienced a powerful fear of hell and an equally strong conviction of her own unworthiness of heaven. Staying with an uncle, a widower who had become a friar in old age, she had read a number of pious books and concluded that the only escape from damnation lay in the earthly purgatory of a convent. For three months she had struggled to convince herself that the trials and distresses of being a nun could not be greater than those of purgatory and I had fully deserved to be in hell. It would not be a great matter to spend my life as though I were in purgatory if afterwards I were to go straight to heaven, which was what I desired. This decision then, to enter the religious life, seems to have been inspired by servile fear more than by love.[7]

No sooner had she forced herself to act on this terrifying logic and enter the convent than her health began to fail.

During her first months in the convent Teresa adjusted to less food, less sleep, less exercise, as well as less warmth in winter and cool in summer than afforded in her father's comfortable home. She weakened quickly and suffered what appears to have been a classic tonic-clonic major epileptic fit. Her affliction might have ended with this one dramatic episode had she not fervently prayed for a prolonged illness as a spiritual exercise. One of the holiest nuns in the convent was an old woman dying slowly from a painful stomach ailment which she bore with great fortitude. Teresa longed to imitate her and endure a similar malady in order to grow in grace. 'I begged God,' she confessed,

> that He would send me any illness He pleased if only He would make me as patient as she. I do not think I was in the least afraid of being ill, for I was so anxious to win eternal blessings that I was resolved to win them by any means whatsoever.[8]

It is reasonable to conjecture that catalepsy followed epilepsy as wish fulfilment: that the psychological condition was an emotional reaction to the depleting convent regime and the epilepsy on the one hand, and to the guilt and explicit yearning for disease on the other. The horrendous medicinal cocktails served by her doctors further complicated her symptoms and increased the organic pathology of her condition.

Two events relieved her crippling anxieties and freed her to walk in an increasingly upright posture. The first was the death of her father in 1543. Cordial relations had been restored between them as soon as Teresa became ill, but an enduring sense of guilt had nevertheless continued to weigh heavily upon her. This seems to have been lifted a year after his death by her resolution to adopt St Joseph as her patron saint.

> I took for my advocate and lord the glorious Saint Joseph and commended myself earnestly to him, and I found that this my father and lord delivered me both from this trouble [i.e. catalepsy] and also from other and greater troubles concerning my honour [i.e. her Jewish heritage] and the loss of my soul [i.e. remorse over disobeying her father and the fear which drove her to the convent], and that he gave me greater blessings than I could ask of him. I do not remember even now that I have ever asked anything of Him which he has failed to grant. I am astonished at the great favours which God has bestowed on me through this blessed saint, and at the perils from which He has freed me, both in body and soul.[9]

She goes on to remind us that St Joseph was our Lord's adopted father; that Jesus obeyed him on earth; and that the risen Christ continues to do as Joseph asks in heaven. She therefore viewed him as a peculiarly potent advocate. Without forcing Teresa into a psychological straightjacket, it is possible to conjecture that with the death of her own father and the adoption of St Joseph, she assuaged her guilt and resolved the emotional problems which largely caused her physical paralysis.

While she was enduring catalepsy, Teresa discovered a means to sustain herself through it and alleviate its pain – prayer. Mercifully for us, she described her prayer life in vivid detail in *The Life, The Way of Perfection, and The Interior Castle*. Teresa was the first woman (and along with Thérèse of Lisieux one of only three) granted the title 'Doctor of the Church'. It is these books which won her this accolade. No one has ever charted the journey of the soul searching for God more thoroughly than she, and no one has ever attempted to do so with such common sense and plain speaking. She believed that it was the mission of every Christian to pray, whatever his or her intelligence, background or education. She recognised prayer not only as the pathway to heaven, but also as the way to bear all of the disappointments, disasters and pains of this life along the way.

For Teresa prayer is the intersection of two forces: the individual disciplining themselves daily to prepare for the divine encounter, and God seizing the initiative to visit how and when he pleases.[10] Preparation entails the pursuit of honesty, charity and humility in relation to God and to other people. This is the essential background to all Christian living, for it satisfies Jesus' basis requirement to 'love the Lord your God with all your heart and all your strength, and your neighbour as yourself'. The fundamental commandment, it is also a dynamic process. As we grow in truth and love, we appreciate with ever-increasing clarity the snares of dishonesty, selfishness and pride. And because these sins are deeply and subtly embedded in the human psyche, we must do regular battle with them to achieve the gradual reformation of character in Jesus' image which prepares mortal human beings more and more fully to meet God.[11]

After embarking on this lifelong quest, Teresa recommends instituting a simple regime of daily solitary prayer. It need not be long but it must be whole-hearted and single-minded. Without any regard to what we might gain immediately or ultimately she bids us to focus our attention on God, letting all distractions pass by without taking notice of them or worrying about them. The easiest way to begin, she tells us, is to say the Lord's Prayer slowly and concentrate fully on each phrase. We may not progress beyond the first phrase or two, but this does not matter. The aim is to understand the whole message of each phrase by exploring its literal meaning and connotations, then savouring its impact on our emotions.[12]

The first words, 'Our Father', for example, invite extended attention, because they define our basic relationship to God. Through Christ we call God 'Father'; through Christ we invite him into our thoughts and lives; and through Christ's example we discover how to conform our aspirations and actions to the *imago Dei*, the hidden, Christlike self within each one of us. Similarly, 'Who art in heaven' offers another fertile image for investigation, because it makes clear that when we are with Christ praying to God, we are already in heaven; and here we can share our pains and stresses and learn how best to handle them. Using this same technique, we can examine different accounts of Jesus' life and teachings in the Bible.

The goal of tackling our sins and practising the simple forms of meditation described by Teresa is the 'prayer of quiet' leading to 'union' with God. We move beyond the state of thinking about a prayer or biblical story; we still our minds; we suspend our thoughts; yet we remain actively attentive to God. This takes practice, but Teresa assures us that if we work diligently at clearing our minds – centring ourselves, as we would say today – we do all in our power to court the Almighty. The rest is up to God, and he is renowned for responding generously.[13] His gifts are fourfold.

The first gift is a deep inner peace which promotes healing. In response to our state of intellectual passivity but emotional alertness, God gives us an intense feeling of calm. Modern scientists inform us that when we enter this realm of peace, our bodies undergo physiological changes: lowered blood pressure, reduced pace of breathing and slower rate of metabolism. The periods of deep physical relaxation experienced in prayer provide respites from the severe tension of pain. A welcome escape in themselves, they also give the body a chance to rest and restore itself by lowering cumulative tension and improving sleep.

The second gift is a reduction in pain. A recent widescale survey of chronic pain-sufferers reveals that eighty per cent reported appreciably lower levels of discomfort once they began regular meditation. This diminution occurs as a result of altered brain functioning. When we pray we advance into a state of being altogether different from ordinary life. With unmoving and seemingly immovable body and with attention riveted on the divine, we seem to float in eternity. As a consequence of physical relaxation and a reduction of the body's general metabolic rate, our brain activity changes. It moves from the low amplitude, high frequency beta waves of normal sharply focused thought to the higher amplitude, lower frequency alpha waves of diffuse, non-analytic slow-moving thought.

The shift in brain activity can be measured on an electro-encephalograph, as amplitude levels rise from a range of one to forty microvolts to a range of forty to seventy microvolts and as the pace of waves diminishes from thirteen cycles per second down to eight. Brain activity slows down even more and amplitude levels rise even higher during periods of 'union with God', when theta waves reach a range of seventy microvolts up to one hundred and the rate slows from eight cycles per second down to four cycles.[14]

Advancing from the alpha to the theta state is a normal pro-gression for those skilled in meditating. Recently, scientists have confirmed that virtually everyone who practises the discipline of daily meditation can learn how to pass from dis-tracted, critical beta patterns to passive alpha ones. In an American study even the most unpromising candidates reached alpha states for eighty-five per cent of their medi-tation time after thirty sessions.[15] The theta mode, which is attainable through persistence in prayer, is celebrated both in religious and scientific literature as the state in which yogis walk on nails and suspend their limbs in near-freezing or boiling water with no discernible pain reaction. Daily medi-tation over many years trains yogis to reduce their response to outside stimuli to a second or two and thus maintain an almost steady level of theta waves, no matter how painful the inter-ruption.[16] Teresa was afforded the same imperturbability through prayer.

Few people can sustain theta waves for as long as a yogi, but Teresa assures us that even the briefest periods of union have profound repercussions. In the early days of her illness, she explains,

> the Lord began to be so gracious to me in this way of prayer that He granted me the favour of leading me to the Prayer of Quiet, and occasionally even to Union, though I did not understand what either of these was, or how highly they were to be valued. It is true that my experience of Union lasted only a short time: I am not sure that it can have been for as long as an Ave Maria [about thirty seconds]; but the results were so considerable, and lasted for so long, that although at the time I was [twenty-three], I seemed to have trampled the world beneath my feet.[17]

Teresa asserts and modern scientists concur that these benefits are the common heritage of all Christians who devote even a half hour every day to meditation.

When brainwaves range between the alpha and theta levels, a healing of the emotions can occur. This is the third gift of prayer. Once the normal flow of thoughts and distractions has been replaced by an observant, passive attitude, we can gaze at ideas and fantasies as they spring to mind but let them go without analysing them. Because our focus is now broad rather than narrow, we cannot cling to a train of thought or an association of daydreams. If disturbing matters cross our mental screens, we surrender them as quickly and easily as pleasant subjects.

It is crucial to remain detached from whatever comes to mind, because over time the kinds of concerns which interrupt our prayers change. At first everyday preoccupations and worries clutter our minds. But as we become skilled at acknowledging and then ignoring these minor irritants, long forgotten and potentially more upsetting material rises to consciousness. This is because many of the seminal emotional experiences which produced these fears and associations occurred during our first five years of childhood, when theta waves predominated. Access to them receded as brain activity accelerated in later childhood and adulthood. In meditation the theta waves of early childhood are replicated and repressed memories become accessible.[18] They rise to consciousness; the mind registers and then releases them; and they become integrated into the fabric of experience.

It is possible that Teresa, herself, found healing in this normal prayer process. Memories of the pain she caused her father as well as the pain she felt at her mother's early death may have been brought to her attention in this dispassionate context, acknowledged, accepted, released and thus vanquished as threats to her wellbeing. Emotional health and maturity may have been provided for her, as for so many others, through the mechanism of disciplined regular prayer.

What is clear and generously documented is that after four years of intense suffering and ten years of gradual improvement, Teresa prayed for a cure and received it. The source of her healing, as she plainly tells us, was divine. But Teresa was not an entirely passive recipient. We know that she made specific requests to God through St Joseph.[19] We also know that entreaties posed in alpha and theta states are far more powerful than petitions made in the beta mode, for they bypass the conscious mind and penetrate to the deepest bedrock of awareness. Repeated often, they actually reprogramme the unconscious mind by forcing it to learn a new response.[20]

In recent years it has been proved in clinical experiments that changes in health and behaviour promoted through meditation are dramatic. Modern doctors recommend creative visualisation centred on an image of health, while Hindus, Buddhists and transcendental meditators suggest mantras repeating a short phrase. Drawing on her own experience, Teresa simply advises the Christian to ponder the Bible assiduously and pray earnestly in preparation for God's healing action.

Gradually and unexpectedly, Teresa received spiritual

healing as the final and greatest benefit of prayer. Over the years, as she became increasingly adept at recollecting herself and finding 'quiet' and 'union', she realised that God was bestowing on her the gift for which all human beings yearn – unconditional love which is deep, abiding and unrestrained. Ever since childhood she had been aware of her love for God, but only in her thirties did she begin to appreciate the immensity of his love for her.[21]

Teresa's realisation of God's love for her was simple yet profound. It had revolutionary consequences. She ceased fretting about her unworthiness of God's attention and began to bask in his acceptance of her, no matter how well she succeeded or how badly she failed at modelling her life on Christ's. Although she continued to battle with sin in order to grow in faith, hope and love, she stopped trying to earn her salvation. Receiving eternal life as pure gift, she experienced the ultimate liberation from the fear of failure, the tyranny of self-criticism and the restricted love of other people. No one but an omnipotent, all-loving God could offer this supreme cure for the human condition.

God did even more than heal Teresa at every level of her being, physically, emotionally and spiritually. He made her a saint. Working on her innermost being, revealed and opened to him during prayer, he transformed her into a luminary of the faith. He achieved this by remoulding her will, making it conform to his will and her own, unique *imago Dei*. As she often reminds us in her writings, she prepared herself for the divine action every day during meditation. As we now appreciate, she did this by stilling her entire being and entering the alpha and then the theta state. In this passive yet receptive attitude she pondered and savoured the prayers of the Church as well as the stories and lessons of the Bible. And, like the petitionary prayers which healed her, these simple words and images reprogrammed her basic will. They led her out of the self-preoccupation of the sick room into God's world of justice, faithfulness, mercy and compassion. In these prayer sessions

God gave her eyes to see the injustice, infidelity and intoler-
ance of her own society and the strength to rectify them. In a
very real sense, he made her a prophet – one who identifies the
sins of God's people and urges them to return to his ways.

From her earliest days in the convent Teresa agonised over
the laxity with which the Carmelite rule was practised in
Spain. She longed to restore its ancient austerity with its commitment to absolute poverty, equality and charity. In 1554 she
rose from her sickbed and began focusing her considerable
determination, courage and leadership skills on founding a
reformed branch of the order. Over the next twenty-eight years
she spent many months doubled-up in a mule cart bumping
across Spain's scorching plain and over icy, barren mountains
to establish seventeen houses of the 'discalced' (barefoot)
Carmelites. Each new convent and monastery was a witness to
the Gospel injunction to sell one's goods, give the proceeds to
the poor and dedicate oneself to a life of service.

Each new foundation was also a personal triumph for
Teresa. In every town she entered there was considerable
opposition to the intrusion of begging friars and nuns drawing
on municipal charities which were already strained by the
unemployed and indigent. Equally, there was opposition to her
insistence that Jewish converts to Christianity be welcomed
into the discalced Carmelites and thus into the wider community.[22] Teresa's obsession with monastic poverty and social
equality contrasted sharply with her contemporaries' dedication to status, honour and conspicuous consumption. Like a
true prophet she insisted that God's laws were superior to
human values and that they must prevail.[23] She displayed
remarkable powers of persuasion in winning local support for
each new venture, in securing royal and episcopal approval
and then in imposing the harsh new discipline on religious
accustomed to a far more lenient regime. But Teresa was an
accomplished diplomat. She knew when to play the humble
submissive woman and when to reveal her will of steel – when
to woo and coax and when to act and speak decisively.

God relieved Teresa of catalepsy and transformed her into a powerful agent of reform, but he did not cure her of all her ills. Like St Paul, she was constantly made weak through physical adversity. Like him, she was daily forced to acknowledge God's strength and her own frailty. Her various maladies not only kept her ever mindful of her dependence on God's grace and favour, they even kept this proud woman humble! Throughout the challenging years on the road Teresa often turned in pain to prayer. Like all of her contemporary religious she suffered the fevers which were an inescapable consequence of communal life, poor sanitation and inadequate nutrition. On one of her numerous journeys across Spain she broke an arm; on another she suffered a stroke and was once again briefly paralysed; on another she experienced a further stroke. Finally, she contracted cancer and died a little more than a year later. In addition to all of this, her doctors diagnosed both heart trouble and consumption (tuberculosis). Intermittent fainting spells testify to the former, but there is little evidence to support the latter.

Taking both Teresa's hyperbolic descriptions and her physicians' questionable diagnoses into account, we must nevertheless conclude that her sixty-seven years were filled with considerable pain and discomfort. Had she not devoted every moment she could spare from travelling, administering and writing to prayer, she might never have recovered from catalepsy or survived her various other afflictions. Through contemplation she found peace with herself and God and mastered her pain. Repeatedly, she unleashed a phenomenal amount of energy to lavish on her mission of monastic reform. Few women have equalled her industry or success in the entire history of Christianity.

Chapter Thirteen

A Path to Eternity

ST TERESA of Avila was an extraordinary woman, but she defined an ordinary path to wholeness. Few Christians become great saints like her, yet all of us are called to live by faith, hope and love and in so doing to transform wherever we are at any particular moment into an outpost of God's kingdom on earth. For many in chronic pain that heavenly citadel is confined to the sickroom. For a few like St Teresa it extends from there to a far wider terrain. Whatever our physical state, contemplative prayer provides the best possible sustenance for this most rewarding of life's labours.

As Teresa warns, learning to still our minds requires much patience and great persistence. As we have seen, American researchers have taught students how they may become still and enter an alpha state in thirty sessions. It appears to have taken Teresa at least five years of daily endeavour to become quietly receptive to God in preparation for the gift of 'union'. It took me closer to twenty years, for my application was less consistent and as a consequence less immediately fruitful. The duration of training is, however, irrelevant because the attainment is worth any amount of effort.

Illness provides an ideal start to this education. Teresa learned the prayer of quiet as she recovered from catalepsy, while I finally discovered the art of stillness after my bout with encephalitis. Such dramatic diseases are most certainly not necessary prerequisites, but they do have the great advantage of removing you from everyday life and its preoccupations for a prolonged period, forcing you into a passive state and only

gradually allowing you to resume normal roles and responsibilities. During the acute phase you are too weak to embark on
any new spiritual exercises, but you are capable of realising a
new sense of time. Prevented from undertaking familiar
activities, you enter a timeless realm. This is an immense boon
and a very useful launching pad to the next stage. As you
regain strength, it becomes possible to preserve this new perception of timelessness. Set the alarm of a nonticking clock for
twenty, thirty or forty minutes; train your attention on stilling
the mind; let thoughts pass unheeded; focus instead on the
void of time and space in which you exist; remain alert to God's
word; and altogether forget the passing moments. Anyone in
chronic pain can seize the inevitable stints of resting in bed to
begin this spiritual enterprise.

Teresa plots a course of prayer from meditation to contemplation which has worked for thousands of Christians over the
past four hundred years. She instructs us to ponder words
from a prayer or short passage from Scripture and to repeat
them again and again until we are completely at peace and
able to enter a quiet world in which time and space are
suspended.

Teresa's method is well worth trying, but it has not worked
for me. This is because words produce both thoughts and
images. Most people can meditate on a passage and then let
the words go, thus quieting their minds yet remaining open to
God in a wordless inner silence. I cannot surrender thoughts,
words and images so freely, as I seem to have a dogged tenacity
in searching for meaning in whatever crosses my mind. For
years this zeal to investigate words and images was an insurmountable obstacle to the prayer of quiet. Through meditation I learned much and hugely enjoyed the experience of
thinking and ruminating, but I did not progress to Teresa's
next stage.

Two keys finally unlocked the door. One was a mantra, a few
words repeated rhythmically. For centuries Indian mystics
have used this simple device to still the mind, and more

recently the transcendental meditation movement has employed it as an aid to relaxation and consciousness-raising. I discovered my mantra in a magnetic resonance imaging machine during a neurological investigation after the encephalitis!

Being claustrophobic, I had for years looked in horror at magazine health insurance advertisements picturing smiling patients being pushed on stretchers into these vast cylinders, and I had long regarded enclosure in such a machine as the worst imaginable form of torture. Now I was the one being strapped into place with my head immobilised in bands of tape. I mentioned claustrophobia to the attending nurse in a voice which I tried to make casual but which clearly betrayed my fear. She responded with total lack of sympathy, briskly ordering me not to move a muscle. Hardly consoling.

As the nurse pushed me headfirst into the cylinder, terror overwhelmed me. I gazed in mounting panic at the 'ceiling' six inches above my eyes. Suddenly, the magnets began making a thunderous noise – three resonating booms followed by a pause and then two more booms. On the brink of hysteria, I realised that it was possible to trace the rhythm of the magnets and inwardly chant 'God is here – keep still' to their ebb and flow. This mantra was my salvation. By repeating it I very quickly entered an alpha state and became impervious to the thudding of the magnets and the agony of containment within the small enclosure. Subsequently, I discovered that this simple mantra could be repeated in unthreatening circumstances to produce the same speedy and beneficial effect.

Why this mantra should work so well during the magnetic resonance imaging investigation and thereafter I do not know, for I had experimented with other mantras over many years to little avail. For months on end I had tried phrases recommended by spiritual giants: the Jesus prayer so favoured by Orthodox Christians ('Lord Jesus Christ, Son of the living God, have mercy on me, a sinner'); the Aramaic mantra of the mystic, John Main ('maranatha'); and simply 'love' (the 'spear' recommended by an anonymous thirteenth-century English mystic to pierce 'the cloud of unknowing'). Experimenting with these mantras must have prepared me for the sudden discovery in the magnetic resonance imaging machine. Its success proves that even the most dedicated of thinkers can – through trial, error and finally gift – enter the realm of quietness.

The second key was physical relaxation. Without it contemplative prayer is, in my experience, impossible. Learning to relax in pain is difficult. Nevertheless, it is essential not simply to pray but more basically to survive. In the first instance this means training yourself to flinch but then relax when a pang assaults. This is a challenge, because over time all of us in chronic pain learn to defend ourselves by anticipating the next searing jab. We become rigid in a posture of frightened expectation. It takes practice to flinch automatically in reaction to pain and then to relax immediately.

By remaining relaxed you achieve two important goals. First, you reduce the duration and intensity of the initial pain sensation. Second, you effectively prepare yourself for subsequent pangs. If you react naturally by retaining your muscles in a taut state, you turn yourself into a board along which pain travels quickly and forcefully. If, however, you relax and transform yourself into a ball of dough, pain passes through you less intensively and extensively. Like finding the right mantra, this may take time. But unless you learn how to relax, you will encounter great difficulty in praying contemplatively while in pain.

My drill is as simple as Teresa's, though slightly different. I sit upright, as kneeling is painful, and in my experience it is essential to find a posture which is balanced and comfortable. Having settled yourself with your back gently – rather than ramrod – straight, breathe deeply and rhythmically and repeat your mantra slowly. With practice you will learn to find the inner world of silence quickly, and there you must wait attentively. You will feel as if you are in eternity, and you will be! You can do no more and must not try, for anything you do will intrude the human world and your own selfhood into the emptiness, thus obstructing access to God. It is he who must take the initiative.

Sometimes a distant experience floats to the surface and then descends again. Let it come and go; ponder both it and its significance later. At other times you will perceive a direct message from God. One of the clearest I have ever received was several months before my mother-in-law's death, when he ordered me to accept her as a person (something I had previously found difficult), to accept the fact that she was dying (something she found difficult) and to hold her hand as she did so. Our relationship was transformed by these commands to me and, I surmise, by other messages imparted to her with equal force and clarity. Our mutual blessing was the discovery of a true love and regard for one another which had eluded us for fifteen years. In my experience most messages are less direct, less rational and far less detailed, but I needed to hear this one fully and unambiguously.

Sometimes God does not respond at all over a long period of time. This is extremely discouraging, yet the challenge is to persevere nevertheless. The attentive waiting does far more than enable us to receive his gifts whenever he chooses to bestow them. It also prepares us for eternity and provides a foretaste of it, for the ultimate and lasting union can only be attained after death.

Contemplative prayer is deeply rewarding, but it is not always possible. Pain can be an impenetrable barrier. If you are in too much pain and are tense, tired and without emotional or physical reserves, then it is a mistake to embark on this kind of prayer. All you will achieve is frustration and disappointment, and a high pain level delivers quite enough of these without the additional burden of failing to remain still, alert and attentive for a reasonable period of time. In such circumstances it is wiser to meditate and intercede for others, keeping your mind occupied for as long as possible, praying

127

through the pain and trying to use the pain creatively rather than avoid it.

In offering this advice I humbly realise that I stand at the foot of the spiritual mountain and that others who have climbed to the top are able to contemplate even in great pain. I very much hope that God will equip me to do the same, but this remains an aspiration for the future rather than a gift currently enjoyed. For the time being contemplation is possible on good days when pain is low and obligations few. Summer holidays and weekend retreats are ideal, and early Sunday mornings are also possible. Though desiring far more, I am greatly consoled by the adage to 'pray as you can, not as you can't'. With this in mind I rejoice that contemplation is possible at least some of the time. I urge all chronic pain sufferers to set out on this most rewarding of ventures as soon as time and pain permit. Contemplative prayer is the ultimate elixir, the 'sovereign remedy to prolong life indefinitely', for it takes one from here to eternity in the ever-passing moment.

Conclusion

Travelling Aids

NO SENSIBLE traveller sets out on a long journey without a kit of travelling aids. The first is usually a map of the unknown terrain ahead. Alas, the uncertainties and imponderables of human existence make it impossible to chart precise paths through pain. I have tried instead to provide a guidebook which identifies the beauty spots and hazards of various routes and which indicates the likely destination of each. I sincerely hope that those in chronic pain find these guides useful in pursuing their own particular paths.

However helpful this handbook may be in pointing out highways, unpaved roads and dead ends, the traveller will create his or her own unique journey. Each of us will follow paths which we find particularly attractive or compelling at different points in our lives. By making these individual choices we decide not only where we shall go, but also who we shall be and become. As St Paul observed from the experience of chronic pain, 'suffering produces endurance, and endurance produces character' (Romans 5:4). Some routes lead us forward in faith, hope and love and promote optimum health of body, emotions and spirit. Others draw us into doubt, frustration and confusion, deplete our capacity to cope with pain and may even add psychological problems to physical ones. The directions we choose are thus of paramount importance.

A second travel aid is a 'rescue remedy' to be used when accidents occur. The best one I have found over many years is a lively sense of humour. It salves frayed nerves like no other medicine. It also boosts the traveller's capacity to surmount obstacles along the road. This is because humour enables us to view problems as objects of amusement rather than as sources of discouragement or causes of disaster. This kind of humour can – and indeed must – be cultivated. It is a function of the will, not a natural ability like the talent for telling a funny story well and making an audience laugh. It is available to everyone, even those like me who cannot tell a joke properly. It relies upon a disciplined effort to maintain a sense of perspective and to develop a delight in the abundant absurdities of life.

Allow me to describe two near disasters which were entirely transformed by humour. The first was the acquisition of a leg brace. My heart plummeted into my toes with my first glimpse at this hideous leather and metal contraption. How, I wondered, could I or anyone else view me as an attractive young woman with this ugly appendage? Indeed how could anyone regard me as anything but a freak? Upon leaving the hospital where it was fitted, I cancelled my plans to attend a barbecue with friends that evening and instead sat alone in my flat with the lights out and my spirits low. The next day I hobbled off to Harvard Square with my head held down and my eyes focused on the pavement. Clearly I presented a figure of considerable pathos. I certainly felt sorry for myself!

Salvation of a most unexpected variety awaited me in the courtyard of the Harvard administration building, where a group of hippies congregated daily to play guitars, entertain passers-by and beg for spare change. Suddenly one of them rushed up to me, bent down, put his face under mine, smiled and enquired: 'Lady, would *you* like some spare change?' Immediately I burst into peals of mirthful laughter, realising how truly pathetic I looked. His humour lifted me out of my misery and buoyed my spirits. I thanked him, returned home, donned a bright yellow dress and hair ribbon and set out again, this time with my head held high and my eyes directly greeting those who gaped in revulsion at the brace.

The friendly hippy taught me that laughter is contagious

and that a smile enables us to feel comfortable with the physically odd and ugly. Perhaps even more importantly, his joke dispelled my own gloom and enabled me to wear this ridiculous object without further concern over my spoiled appearance.

A second near disaster occurred several months later on a train between Brussels and Louvain. Although I had secured the assistance of a porter at the Brussels railway station when boarding the train, I anticipated that none would be available at a little town like Louvain to assist my departure. Burdened with two heavy suitcases and a flight bag – none of which I could manage on crutches – I asked nearby passengers if any would help me get the cases off the train when we reached Louvain. Dead silence. I tried again in French. Dead silence once more, this time etched in frost. ' Wonderful,' I thought. 'Here I am in Flanders with no one willing to speak French or English. What am I to do?' The only apparent solution was to pull down the window and hurl the bags onto the station platform. The vision of this antic instantly reduced me to helpless giggles.

As the train slowed down and I seized the first case, someone shouted 'Attendez' from the end of the carriage and two teenagers advanced to help. Not only did they seize my bags; they also alerted the conductor to the problem and asked him to keep the train in the station until they had found me a cab. All three of us had a good laugh over the frigid display of Flemish nationalism, and I lost all fear of travelling around the world with four legs and no hands. Once again humour had cast out fear and assisted me metaphorically to 'leap' over an insurmountable obstacle.

In the years since then innumerable other occasions have been redeemed by humour. Gradually, I have begun to appreciate the paramount importance of praying for the grace to keep a sense of perspective when pain, events and emotions conspire to lead me into a slough of despondency. Humour depends upon distancing yourself from difficulties which

131

threaten to overwhelm you and then finding something to laugh about. Initially this prayer is uttered as an arid, intellectual exercise, unaccompanied by any speedy lightening of the emotional burden. It begins as an act of will, an articulation of the urgent need for help in discovering a vantage point apart from the mire of troubles. Its blessing is the capacity to stand back a little from the problems, pressures, work and pain and begin to examine them one by one. This prayer helps me to prioritise responsibilities and organise essential rest and recreation. If the pain is bad and the problems are both numerous and complicated, the liberating process can take a seeming eternity. Nevertheless, with tenacity and grace perspective can be gained and humour wrenched from most predicaments.

Over time I am very slowly learning to identify fatigue, overwork and mounting pain early and avoid plunging thoughtlessly into a crisis. Yet even if I remain blind to the lunacy of allowing obligations and pain to mount, my husband will often physically stop me, hold me, ask me to slow down and get me to laugh at my whirling dervish gyrations. This is not to say that either one of us trivialises pain or real life problems, rather that we are becoming ever more adept at viewing them sensibly and appreciating that we should laugh about as many as possible as frequently as possible. The alternative is to allow ourselves to slide into a pit of despair from which escape would be harder and harder over time as pain increases and problems accumulate.

The third and most important travel aid is faith – faith that the journey is worthwhile, faith that even wrong turns are instructive and useful, faith that there is something to discover and some way to grow in hope and love at every point along the way right to the end. Faith comes to the rescue when knowledge fails. It lifts the traveller's gaze above immediate pain and distress. It incorporates present, past and future suffering into a vision of ultimate wholeness, into a world made perfect beyond the scope of our earthly lives and limited human understanding. Faith inspires us to offer ourselves, our souls, our bodies and our pain to God so that he can redeem us and the universe in ways we cannot begin to imagine. It enables us to respect the mystery enshrouding pain and life itself and affirm with St Julian of Norwich, a fellow traveller on the paths through pain, that 'all shall be well, and all shall be well, and all manner of things shall be well'.

Notes

Chapter One: My Itinerary

1. The phrase 'slow, silent revolution' was used by R. W. Southern in his *Making of the Middle Ages* (New Haven, Yale University Press, 1968) to describe changes occurring in early medieval society, gradually and almost imperceptibly creating new cultural, social, economic and political forms in Western Europe. These memorable words admirably describe the nature and timing of the individual sufferer's move from denial through acceptance to living creatively with pain. The transition is of monumental importance, but it does not occur swiftly or ostentatiously.
2. Elisabeth Kübler-Ross, *On Death and Dying* (New York, Macmillan, 1969).

Chapter Two: The Straight Road to Heaven

1. *The Acts of the Christian Martyrs*, trans. by Herbert Musurillo (Oxford, Clarendon Press, 1972), p. 3.
2. Herbert Workman, *The Martyrs of the Early Church* (London, Charles Kelly, 1913), pp. 109ff.
3. Musurillo, pp. xxv–xxvi.
4. ibid., pp. 109–15.
5. Chris Jones, 'Women, Death and the Law During the Christian Persecutions', in Diana Wood (ed.), *Martyrs and Martyrologies* (Oxford, Blackwell Publishers for the Ecclesiastical History Society, 1993), p. 26.
6. Musurillo, pp. 127–31.
7. ibid., p. 35.
8. ibid., pp. 302–9.

9. Elizabeth Rundle, *Martyrs and Saints of the First Twelve Centuries* (London, SPCK, 1910), pp. 166–8.

10. ibid., pp. 175–6.

11. ibid., pp. 173–4.

12. Musurillo, pp. 132–5.

13. Revelation 7:9–10, 13–17.

Chapter Four: The Holy Highway

1. See Dom Cuthbert Butler (ed.), *The Rule of St Benedict* (Collegeville Minnesota, Liturgical Press, 1948).

2. Jean LeClercq, *The Love of Learning and the Desire for God* (New York, The New American Library of World Literature, 1962), pp. 38–40.

3. Thomas à Kempis, *The Imitation of Christ* (London, Hodder and Stoughton, 1979), Book One, ch. 25, p. 62.

4. ibid., Book One, ch. 17, p. 41.

5. ibid., Book One, ch. 22, p. 52.

6. ibid., Book Two, ch. 38, p. 75.

7. Sandra M. Schneiders IHM, 'Contemporary Religious Life: Death or Transition?', in Cassian Yuhaus (ed.), *The Challenge for Tomorrow's Religious Life* (New York, The Paulist Press, 1994), p. 10.

8. Lawrence Cada (ed.), *Shaping the Coming Age of Religious Life* (New York, The Seabury Press, 1979), pp. 14–50.

9. ibid., p. 30.

10. ibid., p. 38.

11. ibid., p. 39.

12. ibid., p. 43.

13. ibid., p. 48.

14. For a broader discussion, see Joan Chittister OB, 'An Amazing Journey: A Road of Twists and Turns', in Yuhaus, pp. 76–91, and also her *Fire in These Ashes* (Kansas City, Sheed and Ward, 1995).

15. Benjamin Tonna STD, 'A Discerning Approach to Contemporary Religious Life', in Cada, pp. 56–7.

Chapter Five: Travelling Tips from Monks and Nuns

1. Almighty God, Father of all Mercies, we thine unworthy servants do give thee most humble and hearty thanks for all thy goodness

and loving kindness to us and to all men [rehearsing here particular thanks for the day just passed]. We bless thee for our creation, preservation and all the blessings of this life; but above all, for the redemption of the world by our Lord, Jesus Christ; for the means of grace and for the hope of glory. And, we beseech thee, give us a due sense of all thy mercies, that our hearts may be unfeignedly thankful, and that we show forth thy praise, not only with our lips, but in our lives; by giving up ourselves to thy service, and by walking before thee in holiness and righteousness all our days; through Jesus Christ our Lord, to whom with thee and the Holy Ghost be all honour and glory, world without end. Amen.

Modern renditions of this prayer are available in the *Alternative Service Book of 1980* in England and the revised *Book of Common Prayer* used by the American Episcopal Church. I prefer the version quoted above and included in the 1928 prayer books in both England and the United States, partly because I grew up with it and partly because I find the language beautiful, congenial and inspiring.

2. Thomas à Kempis, *The Imitation of Christ* (London, Hodder and Stoughton, 1979) Book One, ch. 21, p. 49.

Chapter Six: The Path that Leads to a Dead End

1. George Widengren, *Mani and Manicheanism* (London, Weidenfeld and Nicholson, 1965), p. 24.
2. ibid., p. 660.
3. ibid., p. 64.
4. ibid., p. 140.
5. Walter Wakefield, *Heresy, Crusade and Inquisition in Southern France, 1100–1250* (London, George Allen and Unwin Ltd, 1974), p. 27.
6. ibid., p. 137.
7. ibid., p. 250.
8. D. M. Walmsey, *Anton Mesmer* (London, Robert Hall, 1967), p. 57.
9. ibid., pp. 135–8.
10. Henry James, *The Bostonians* (London, The Bodley Head, 1967), p. 60.
11. Before embarking on Mrs Eddy's fascinating story, I must point out the hazards of gathering information and drawing conclusions about a woman who is revered as the greatest woman in history

by her most ardent followers, yet damned as a dictatorial charla-
tan by disenchanted members of the Christian Science Church.
The pens of her biographers have been dipped either in liquid gold
or in venom! Reconciling evidence of her sanctity on the one hand
and her deranged zealotry on the other has posed a considerable
challenge. I hope that what follows is a balanced account of this
remarkable woman's life.

12. Edward Franden Dakin, *Mrs Eddy* (New York, Blue Ribbon
Books, 1930), p. 19.
13. John Haller, 'Neurasthenia: The Medical Profession and the "New
Woman" of the Late Nineteenth Century', *New York Journal of
Medicine* (12 February 1971), pp. 473–84.
14. Dakin, p. 503.
15. E. Mary Ramsay, *Christian Science and Its Discoverer* (Boston,
Massachusetts, The Christian Science Publishing Society, 1935),
p. 20.
16. ibid., p. 44.
17. Robert Peel, *Mary Baker Eddy* (Boston, Massachusetts, The
Christian Science Publishing Society, 1971), vol. II, p. 125.
18. R. Lawrence Moore, *Religious Outsiders and the Making of
Americans* (Oxford, Oxford University Press, 1986), p. 33.
19. ibid., p. 125.
20. ibid., p. 75.
21. ibid., p. 52.
22. Dakin, p. 125.
23. ibid., p. 112.
24. Peel, vol. III, p. 354.
25. Dakin, p. 123.
26. ibid., p. 506.
27. Caroline Fraser, 'Suffering Children and the Christian Science
Church', *The Atlantic Monthly* (April 1995), p. 108.
28. ibid., p. 113.

Chapter Eight: **A Road to Disaster**

1. Richard Friedman, 'The Depressed Masochistic Patient:
Diagnostic and Management Considerations – A Contemporary
Psychoanalytic Perspective', in *Journal of the American Academy
of Psychoanalysis* (1991), vol. 19 (1), p. 12.
2. Quoted by Jack Novick and Kerry Kelly Novick, 'Some Comments

on Masochism and the Delusion of Omnipotence from a Developmental Perspective', *Journal of the American Psychoanalytic Association* (1991), vol. 39 (2), p. 307.

3. Sigmund Freud, 'The Economic Problem of Masochism', in *Collected Papers, Clinical Papers* (The International Psycho-Analytical Library, London, 1924), vol. II, pp. 255–68.

4. *The Dictionary and Statistical Manual of Mental Disorder III Revised (DSM III–R)* 3rd edn (American Psychiatric Association, Washington DC, 1987), p. 373.

5. Suzanne Lego, 'Masochism: Implications for Psychiatric Nursing', *Archives of Psychiatric Nursing* (August 1992), vol. VI, no. 4, pp. 225–9.

6. Cheryl Glickauf-Hughes and Marilyn Wells, 'Current Conceptualizations on Masochism: Genesis and Object Relation', *American Journal of Psychotherapy* (January 1991), vol. XLV, no. 1, p. 57.

7. *The Dictionary and Statistical Manual of Mental Disorder IV Revised (DSM IV–R)* 4th edn (American Psychiatric Association, Washington DC, 1994), pp. 373–4.

8. Friedman, pp. 19–29.

9. A. H. Crisp, 'The Psychopathology of Anorexia Nervosa: Getting the "Heat" out of the System', in Albert J. Stunkard and Eliot Stellar (eds.), *Eating and Its Disorders* (Raven Press, New York, 1984), p. 209.

10. ibid., pp. 216–7.

11. Paul E. Garfinkel and David M. Garner, 'The Multidetermined Nature of Anorexia Nervosa', in Padraig L. Darby, Paul E. Garfinkel, David M. Garner and Donald Corsina, *Anorexia Nervosa: Recent Developments in Research* (New York, Alan R. Liss, Inc., 1983), p. 9.

12. David M. Garner, Paul E. Garfinkel and Marion P. Olsted, 'An Overview of Sociocultural Factors in the Development of Anorexia Nervosa', in Darby, Garfinkel *et al.*, p. 66.

13. Vivian Rakoff, 'Multiple Determinants of Family Dynamics in Anorexia Nervosa', in Darby, Garfinkel *et al.*, pp. 30–1.

14. Paul E. Garfinkel and David M. Garner, 'The Multidetermined Nature of Anorexia Nervosa', in Darby, Garfinkel *et al.*, p. 6.

15. Rakoff, 'Multiple Determinants of Family Dynamics in Anorexia Nervosa', in Darby, Garfinkel *et al.*, p. 31.

16. ibid., pp. 32–3.

139

17. Donald M. Schwartz, Michael G. Thompson and Craig L. Johnson, 'Eating Disorders and the Culture', in Darby, Garfinkel *et al.*, pp. 83–4.
18. Rakoff, 'Multiple Determinants of Family Dynamics in Anorexia Nervosa', in Darby, Garfinkel *et al.*, p. 38.
19. *DSM IV–R*, pp. 539–41.
20. Garfinkel and Garner, 'The Multidetermined Nature of Anorexia Nervosa', in Darby, Garfinkel *et al.*, pp. 4–5.
21. Crisp, pp. 211–5.
22. Rudolf Bell, *Holy Anorexia* (London, University of Chicago Press, 1985), p. 19.
23. ibid., pp. 20–1.
24. Blessed Raymond of Capua, *The Life of St Catherine of Siena*, trans. by George Lamb (London, Harvill Press, 1960), p. 22.
25. Arrigo Levassti, *My Servant, Catherine*, trans. by Dorothy White (London, Blackfriars Publications, 1954), p. 5.
26. Raymond of Capua, pp. 40–1.
27. Bell, p. 40.
28. Raymond of Capua, pp. 42, 53 and 54.
29. ibid., p. 38.
30. ibid., p. 376.
31. Levassti, p. 353.
32. Bell, p. 53.
33. Caroline Walker Bynum, *Holy Feasts and Holy Fasts: The Religious Significance of Food to Medieval Women* (London, University of California Press, 1987), p. 6.
34. ibid., p. 30.
35. ibid., p. 170.
36. ibid., p. 171.
37. Donald Wernstein and Rudolf Bell, *Saints and Society: The Two Worlds of Western Christendom, 1000–1700* (London, University of Chicago Press, 1982), p. 234. See also Bell, Table 3, pp. 176–7.

Chapter Ten: St Thérèse of Lisieux's 'Little Way'

1. Brother Bernard Bro, *The Little Way* (London, Darton, Longman & Todd, 1979), pp. 3, 8.
2. ibid., p. 4.

3. St Thérèse of Lisieux, *Autobiography of a Saint*, trans. by Ronald Knox (London, The Harvill Press, 1958), p. 38.
4. Ida Friederike Gorres, *The Hidden Face: A Study of St Thérèse of Lisieux* (London, Burns and Oates, 1959), p. 44.
5. St Thérèse, p. 98.
6. Bro, p. 4.
7. ibid., p. 8.
8. Gorres, p. 49.
9. St Thérèse, p. 83.
10. Gorres, p. 79.
11. St Thérèse, p. 93.
12. ibid., pp. 169–70.
13. ibid., p. 172.
14. ibid., pp. 127–8.
15. ibid., see pp. 153–4, 188, 197, 218 and 268.
16. ibid., p. 186.
17. ibid., p. 186.
18. Thomas à Kempis, *The Imitation of Christ* (London, Hodder and Stoughton, 1979) Book 3, ch. 19, p. 118.
19. St Thérèse, p. 192.
20. ibid., p. 193.
21. ibid., p. 188.
22. ibid., p. 188.
23. ibid., p. 248.
24. St Francis de Sales, *Introduction to the Devout Life* (Image Books, New York, 1972), pp. 121–8.
25. ibid., pp. 39–40.
26. St Thérèse, p. 311.
27. ibid., p. 237.
28. George Herbert, 'Easter', *A Choice of George Herbert's Verse* (London, Faber and Faber, 1967) pp. 24–5.
29. St Thérèse, p. 294.
30. ibid., p. 294.
31. ibid., p. 296.
32. ibid., p. 299.
33. ibid., p. 185.
34. ibid., pp. 129–30.
35. ibid., p. 261.
36. Gorres, p. 3.
37. St Thérèse, pp. 184-5.

38. ibid., p. 252.
39. Etienne Obo, *Two Portraits of St Teresa of Lisieux* (London, 1955), p. 152.
40. Bro, p. 11.
41. ibid., p. 11.
42. ibid., p. 54.
43. ibid., pp. 255–6.
44. ibid., p. 257.
45. Benedict Williamson, *The Victim State* (London, Alexander Ouseley Ltd, 1938), p. 106.
46. ibid., p. 114.

Chapter Eleven: Steps Through the Passing Moment

1. E. M. Blaiklock (ed.), *The Practice of the Presence of God* (London, Hodder and Stoughton, 1993), p. 13.
2. ibid., p. 23.
3. ibid., p. 23.
4. ibid., p. 25.
5. ibid., p. 28.
6. ibid., p. 41.
7. ibid., p. 38.
8. ibid., p. 60.
9. ibid., p. 91.
10. W. H. Auden (ed.), *George Herbert* (London, Penguin Books, 1973), p. 116.
11. Robert B. Shaw, *The Call of George Herbert: The Theme of Vocation in the Poetry of Donne and Herbert* (Boston, Massachusetts, Cowley Publications, 1981), p. 85.
12. ibid., p. 86.
13. Jean-François Six, *Light of the Night: The Last Eighteen Months in the Life of Thérèse of Lisieux* (London, SCM Press Ltd, 1996), p. 49.

Chapter Twelve: St Teresa of Avila's Great Way

1. Rowan Williams, *Teresa of Avila* (London, Geoffrey Chapman, 1991), p. 13.
2. The events of Teresa's life are summarised by E. Allison Peers (trans. and ed.), *The Complete Works of St. Teresa* (London, Sheed

and Ward, 1975), vol. I, pp. xxvi–xxxv, and are vividly described by Teresa herself, in the 'Life', which constitutes vol. I of *The Complete Works*.

3. ibid., vol. I, p. 32.
4. ibid., vol. I, p. 32.
5. ibid., vol. I, pp. 29–30.
6. ibid., vol. I, p. 20.
7. ibid., vol. I, p. 19.
8. ibid., vol. I, p. 27.
9. ibid., vol. I, pp. 34–5.
10. ibid., vol. II, pp. 88–182.
11. ibid., vol. II, p. 64.
12. ibid., vol. II, pp. 90–7.
13. ibid., vol. II, pp. 126–40.
14. Jonathan D. Cowan, Ph.D, 'Alpha-Theta Brainwave Biofeedback: The Many Possible Theoretical Reasons for Its Success', *Biofeedback* (June 1993), p. 12.
15. Joe Kamiya, 'Operant Control of the EEG Alpha Rhythm and Some of its Reported Effects on Consciousness' in Charles T. Tait, *Altered States of Consciousness* (New York and London, John Wiley and Sons Inc., 1969), p. 515.
16. B. K. Anand, G. S. Chhina and Baldev Singh, 'Some Aspects of Electroencephalographic Studies in Yogis' in Tait, p. 505.
17. Peers, vol. I, p. 23.
18. Cowan, p. 15.
19. Peers, vol. l, p. 36.
20. Cowan, p. 14.
21. See Rowan Williams, pp. 52–4, for a more detailed explanation of the theme.
22. ibid., p. 18.
23. ibid., p. 24.

Index